PT Exam Review

The Essential Guide for
the Foreign-Trained
Physical Therapist

PT Exam Review

The Essential Guide for
the Foreign-Trained
Physical Therapist

Iwona Korzeniowska, PT
Rick Schnoll, MA
Aneta Tomaszkiewicz, MA

Publisher: John H. Bond
Acquisitions Editor: Amy E. Drummond
Production Editor: Debra L. Clarke
Art Director: Linda Baker

Printed in the United States of America

Published by: SLACK Incorporated
6900 Grove Road
Thorofare, NJ 08086-9447 USA
Telephone: (609) 848-1000
Fax: (609) 853-5991

Contact SLACK Incorporated for further information about other books in this field or about the availability of our books from distributors outside the United States.

Last digit is print number: 10 9 8 7 6 5 4 3 2 1

Contents

Introduction

This book is designed to help **foreign-trained** physical therapists, living in either another country or in the United States, pass the national licensing examination, obtain a visa and license, and get a good job working as a physical therapist in America.

As you are probably already aware, working and living in the United States can be a difficult thing to accomplish for a foreign-trained professional due to all of the necessary paperwork and procedures. If you are unfamiliar with the American system, this task may seem impossible to do alone. For this reason, many foreign-trained PTs pay thousands of dollars to a "professional" person who only has the information you need to do the same thing **yourself**.

In this book, we will show you step by step how to get a license and a visa to work as a physical therapist in any state in America. We will also give some helpful tips and information for getting the job of your choice. In addition, this book will explain how to get permanent residence status (a "green card") once you are working as a licensed PT.

In order to work as a foreign-trained PT in America you must complete all of the necessary paperwork. The most difficult part for most foreign PTs, however, is in passing the national licensing examination. Because you may be unfamiliar with the way this exam is written, we have devoted the majority of this book to helping you prepare for this exam. We will show you how the exam is structured, what material will be tested, what you should study, and what kinds of techniques you should use while taking the test. This book will also help you with the English language, which we believe is necessary for success in the examination.

We wish you the best of luck in becoming one of the many successful foreign-trained physical therapists working and living in the United States.

Chapter 1
How to Obtain a Physical Therapy License

Every physical therapist who is working in America **must** have a license if he or she wants to practice physical therapy in America. This is true for American as well as foreign therapists. This chapter will explain everything you need to know to obtain a physical therapy license in America.

Useful Terminology

Before we can explain what you need to do, there are a few concepts which you need to understand. Here are the most important ones:

State Licensing Board

Each state has an organization that decides whether to allow you to practice as a physical therapist in America. Each of the 50 states has its own licensing board of physical therapy. It is important to understand that *each state has different requirements for issuing a license*. You must also remember that any information provided in this book may have changed since the last printing, since states do sometimes change their requirements. When you contact the licensing board of the state in which you are interested in working, they will let you know exactly what the requirements are at that time.

National Licensing Examination

This is the most difficult area for foreign-trained physical therapists. In order to get a license in any state, the state will require that you (and American therapists as well) have a certain score on the national licensing exam. The PES (Professional Examination Service) is the company that organizes and gives the results of this exam. The exam is given in each state on the same day, usually three (some states only 1 or 2) times per year (March, July, and November). On any given test date (for example, July 13, 1995) the exam will be *exactly* the same all over the country. The number of questions you must answer correctly to get your license, however, is different in each state. Again, because changes are constantly being made, it is impossible to provide the numbers here.

What does **not** change, though, is the structure of the exam. You will have four hours (3 hours for PTAs) to complete 200 (150 for PTAs) multiple choice questions (A, B, C, or D) that will cover a wide variety of topics in physical therapy. While most of the questions deal with actual knowledge of practicing therapy, there are quite a few questions that have to do specifically with the American healthcare system. This is one of the difficulties facing foreign-trained PTs. Questions about insurance, legal issues, ethics, and administration are common. The other difficulty for foreign PTs, of course, is that the exam is in English. The level of your English will directly influence your success on this exam.

Credentials Evaluation

Because you graduated from a physical therapy program in another country, before you can be issued a license in some states you must have your credentials evaluated. This means that someone must look closely at all of the courses that you studied at the university and also see your diploma and license (if you have a license in your country). There are only a few companies in America that perform this kind of service, and each state accepts an evaluation from different companies. When you apply to a state for a license, they will give you information about which companies you can use for your credentials evaluation.

You will also be instructed about which documents you will have to provide. Usually, the company will want either a notarized copy or the original copy of your diploma of graduation, license, and course transcripts. Once you contact a state, they will tell you exactly what they require.

You should also be aware that the documents just mentioned (diploma, license, transcripts) will usually have to be sent to the state licensing board as well as to the credentials evaluation company. They may also require a photo identification and letters of recommendation from employers or professors. Again, you will be told exactly what you must provide.

Important: When sending a group of documents to any organization or state board, be sure to send all documents **together**. Do not send your diploma one day and your transcripts a week later. Send all of the documents together in the same envelope.

Temporary License/Permanent License

A permanent license is what you must have to be a fully registered, practicing physical therapist in a particular state in America. In addition to a permanent license, however, there is something called a temporary license, and this is very important to a foreign-trained physical therapist.

A temporary license allows you to work as a therapist in the United States (under a licensed therapist's supervision) until you have taken the PES national licensing exam. Depending on which state and when you apply for the temporary license, it can be valid for as long as a year or more. Usually, however, a license is good for a period of six months or until the results of the exam are released.

Not every state issues temporary licenses, but you can check the chart on this page to see which states do. We **strongly** recommend that you choose to work in a state that issues temporary licenses-- especially if you are coming directly from another country. There are two big reasons for this. First, you will have the opportunity to work in a facility and become familiar with the American healthcare system, which can give you useful information for the exam. Second, you will be able to work and earn enough money to live comfortably while you are studying and preparing to take the examination. We will have a final suggestion regarding temporary licenses at the end of this chapter.

TOEFL, TSE, TWE, and TOEIC tests

Educational and licensing institutions in the United States recognize these English tests as good indicators of a foreign person's level of English proficiency. Some states will require that you take one or more of these tests and get a high enough score before they will issue you a temporary or permanent license (see chart). Some of these tests can be taken in your home country, but you may have to come to the United States in some cases. Each of these tests is slightly different and measures a different aspect of English ability. Here is more information about each, as well as the number you can call to find out where the test is being offered.

TOEFL- (Test Of English as a Foreign Language) (609) 951-1100. This is by far the most common and recognized English language test around the world. It consists of three sections: Listening Comprehension, Structure and Written Expression, and Vocabulary and Reading Comprehension.

TSE- (Test of Spoken English) (609) 951-1100. This test specifically measures your ability to speak English. There are a variety of exercises that all require you to speak into a tape recorder for later evaluation.

TWE- (Test of Written English) (609) 951-1100. This test specifically measures your ability to write in English. The test requires that you write an essay which shows your ability to generate and organize your ideas, support them with examples or evidence, and respond to the assigned topic.

TOEIC- (Test Of English for International Communication) (609) 951-1600. This test is similar in format to the TOEFL.

State-by-State Requirements

Here is a chart that lists each state's policy regarding temporary licenses and English tests:

STATE	TEMPORARY LICENSE	ENGLISH TEST	CREDENTIALS EVALUATION
ALA.	N	Y	Y
ALASKA*	N	N	Y
ARIZ.	Y	N	Y
ARK.	N	Y	Y
CALIF.	N	N	Y
COLO.	Y	N	N
CONN.	Y	N	Y
DEL.	Y	N	Y
FLA.	Y	N	Y
GA.	Y	Y	Y
HAWAII	Y	Y	Y
IDAHO	N	N	Y
ILL.	Y	N	N**
IND.	Y	N	Y
IOWA	Y	N	Y
KANSAS	Y	Y	Y
KY.	Y	Y	Y
LA.	Y	Y	Y
MAINE***	Y	Y	Y
MD.	Y	Y	Y
MASS.	Y	Y	Y
MICH.	Y	Y	Y
MINN.	Y	Y	Y
MISS.	Y	Y	Y
MONT.	Y	Y	Y
NEB.	Y	Y	Y
NEV.	Y	Y	Y
N.H.	Y	Y	Y
N.J.	Y	Y	Y
N.M.	Y	N	Y
N.Y.	Y	N	Y

N.C.	N	Y	Y
N.D.	Y	Y	Y
OHIO	N	Y	Y
OKLA.	Y	N	Y
ORE.	Y	N	Y
PA.	N	N	Y
R.I.	N	Y	Y
S.C.	Y****	Y	Y
S.D.	N	N	Y
TENN.	Y	N	Y
TEXAS	Y	N	Y
UTAH	N	N	Y
VT.	Y	N	Y
VA.*	N	Y	Y
WASH.	N	Y	Y
WASH. D.C.	N/A	N/A	N/A
W.VA.	Y	N	Y
WISC.	Y	Y	Y
WYO.	Y	Y	Y

* Must complete 6 month in state internship period before application for exam

** Individual program must be approved

*** Must have at least 6 months work experience as a PT

**** Only for new graduates

Step-by-Step Application Procedure

Now that you are familiar with some of the important concepts, you can follow this step by step guide to getting your license.

Step 1: *Make sure that the physical therapy program that you attended was a **four-year program** (two-year program for PTA).* This is very important. If you studied at a university that had only a three-year PT program, the **only** states that you can possibly work in are Michigan, Illinois, and New York.

Step 2: *Determine your level of English.* This may not be an easy thing to do. You may not be able to accurately judge exactly how good your English is. Obviously, if you speak absolutely no English, you would have an impossible time trying to find a job in the United States (and a difficult time trying to read this book). If you are very sure that your English is not good enough to pass any tests, you should probably consider choosing a state that does not require any English scores.

Step 3: *Choose a state that issues a temporary license.* Again, we must emphasize that it is much easier to come to the United States and work as a therapist while preparing for the exam, rather than simply arriving two weeks before the test. Even if you are already in the United States, it will be helpful to work in a facility to learn more about the system.

Step 4: *Contact the state and request an application.* When asking for an application, be sure to specify that you wish to get your license by **exam**, not by **endorsement** (we will explain endorsement shortly). Also, ask how many times per year the exam is given, to determine how long your temporary license will be valid. You can contact the state by phone or mail. The numbers and addresses can be found at the end of this chapter.

Step 5: *Follow the instructions of the application.* Remember, each state has slightly different requirements, such as whether to send originals or copies, which documents to send, etc. It is extremely important to follow the instructions **exactly**, because any mistakes will cause long delays in the process and you may miss the deadline for the next exam (we will explain more about the deadlines for application later).

Step 6: *Begin your job search.* This is an essential step, because you cannot get a working visa without already having a job. Chapter 2 will give you helpful information about finding a job as a physical therapist in the United States.

Further Points

There are two more terms which you should also be familiar with:

Letter of Supervision: All states which issue a temporary license require that you be supervised at all times by a licensed PT while treating patients. Some states, however, will require a **letter of supervision** signed by a licensed therapist who will be supervising you at your future job.

When you get your application form and it requires a letter of supervision, you must have a job first before they can issue you a temporary license. This does not mean you can't complete the application process and be registered to take the national exam. When you later find a job, the letter of supervision will be sent directly from your employer to the state licensing board.

License By Endorsement: This applies to a physical therapist who is already fully licensed in one state but wishes to transfer his or her license to another state. Again, a credentials evaluation is still needed, along with whatever documents that particular state requires.

Important: When deciding when to apply for a temporary license, it is important to find out when the deadline (final date) is for submitting your application and registering for the upcoming examination. In most states the temporary license is only valid until the results of the national exam you have taken are available. Beacause you want to have the longest possible time to work on a temporary license, it is best to send in your application materials the day **after** the deadline, so that you are registered to take the **following** exam.

For example, suppose the examination is given on July 13, 1995 (and the results are returned around the end of August) with the deadline for registration on June 1, 1995. If you submit all of your application materials on May 28, 1995, your temporary license will only be valid approximately 2-3 months. If, however, you submit your materials on June 3, 1995, you will be registered to take the November 1995 exam (with results due around January 1996). Now your temporary license will be valid 7-8 months, which gives you more time to work and prepare for the exam.

If You Fail the Examination

One final question remains. What do you do if you have failed the national licensing examination? Well, obviously this is not a good situation, however, all hope is not lost. There are still several things you can do.

If you have failed but you had a high score (close to passing), you can still possibly get a permanent license in another state by **transferring** your score to a state that has a lower requirement (remember that each state sets its own passing score). First, you must call the different states to find out if your score might be considered passing. Ask them whether the score for their state is lower than the score for your state. If it is much lower, you must next call PES (Professional Examination Services) at (212) 870-2724 and request an **application for transfer of scores** to be sent to you.

If you wish to make the process go faster, you can write PES a letter stating that you are requesting a transfer of your exam score to the state you are choosing. They will need the following information: Your first and last name, your social security number (you will get one when you come to the United States), the date, month, and year when the exam was taken, the state in which you took the exam, and the exam identification number. If you are not sure of the identification number, you can call the state licensing board in the state where you took the exam. Send this information, along with a check for $40 ($20 if this is your second time) to:

PES
475 Riverside Dr.
New York, NY 10115

Another possibility that you might consider if you have failed the exam by 1 or 2 points is to pay $50 and have your exam scored by hand rather than by computer. At times the computer can make a mistake, possibly by picking up an unintentional pencil mark. If you have come that close to passing, it is probably worth spending the $50 to try (this must be done within 90 days of the results). For this you must also contact PES at (212) 870-3173. You can write to them at the same address, but address the envelope to PES Statistics Department.

The final thing that can be done is to wait for the next exam and try it again. As long as your working visa is still valid, you can legally remain in the country (but you cannot work). The working visa is valid for different amounts of time, depending on the length of the contract you have made with your employer (see Chapters 2 and 3).

State Phone Numbers and Addresses

Alabama
AL Board of PT
400 S. Union St.
Suite 315
Montgomery, AL 36130
(205) 242-4064

Alaska
Licensing Examiner
Therapy Board
P.O. Box 110806
Juneau, AK 99811-0806
(907) 465-2551

Arizona
AZ State Board of
PT Examination
1645 W. Jefferson,
Suite 410
Phoenix, AZ 85007
(602) 542-3095

Arkansas
AR State Board of PT
3 Financial Ctre., Suite 300
Little Rock, AR 72211
(501) 228-7100

California
PT Examining Committee
1434 Howe Ave., Suite 92
Sacramento, CA 95825
(916) 263-2550

Colorado
PT Registration
1560 Broadway, Suite 670
Denver, CO 80202
(303) 894-2440

Connecticut
Dept. of Health Services-
PT License
150 Washington St.
Hartford, CT 06106
(203) 566-1042

Delaware
Division of Professional
Regulation
P.O. Box 1401
Dover, DE 19903
(302) 739-4522

District of Columbia
D.C. Board of PT
614 H Street NW
9th Floor-Rm. 923
Washington, DC 20001
(202) 727-7454

Florida
Dept. of Professional
Regulation
1940 N. Monroe St.
Tallahassee, FL 32399
~~(904) 487-3372~~

Georgia
GA State Board of PT-
State Examining Boards
166 Pryor St., SW
Atlanta, GA 30303
(404) 656-3921

Hawaii
Board of PT
1010 Richards St.
Honolulu, HI 96813
(808) 586-2696

Idaho
ID Board of Medicine
280 N. 8th St., Suite 202
Boise, ID 83720
(208) 334-2822

Illinois
Dept. of Professional
Regulation
320 W. Washington St.,
3rd Floor
Springfield, IL 62786
(217) 782-8556

Indiana
Health Profession Bureau
402 W. Washington St.
Room 041
Indianapolis, IN 46204
(317) 232-2960

Iowa
Board of PT- Dept. of
Public Health
4th Floor Lucas Bldg.
Des Moines, IA 50319
(515) 281-7074

Kansas
KS State Board of
Healing Arts
235 SW Topeka Blvd.
Topeka, KS 66603
(913) 296-7413

Kentucky
KY State Board of PT
9110 Leesgate Rd., Suite 6
Louisville, KY 40222
(502) 595-4687

Louisiana
LA State Board of PT
Examiners
2014 Pinhook Rd.,
Suite 701
Lafayette, LA 70508
(318) 262-1043

Maine
Board of Examiners in PT
State House Station
Number 35
Augusta, ME 04333
(207) 782-8723

Maryland
Board of PT Examiners
4201 Peterson Ave.,
No. 316
Baltimore, MD 21215
(410) 764-4752

Massachussetts
Board of Allied Health
100 Cambridge St.
Room 1516
Boston, MA 02202
(617) 727-3071

Michigan
Dept. of Commerce
BOPR/Health Services
P.O. Box 30018
Lansing, MI 48909
(517) 335-0930

Minnesota
Board of Med Practice
2700 University Ave. W,
Suite106
St. Paul, MN 55114-1080
(612) 642- 0538

Mississippi
MS State Dept. of
Health-Licensure Division
P.O. Box 1700
Jackson, MS 39215
(610) 987-4153

Missouri
MO Board of Healing Arts
P.O. Box 4
Jefferson City, MO 65102
(314) 751-0144

Montana
Dept. of Commerce-
Board of PT Examiners
P.O. Box 200513
11 N. Jackson
Helena, MT 59620-0513
(406) 444-3728

Nebraska
Dept. of Health- Bureau of
Exam Boards
P.O. Box 95007
301 Centennial Mall S.
Lincoln, NE 68509-5007
(402) 471-2115

Nevada
Nevada State Board of
Examiners
P.O. Box 81467
Las Vegas, NV 89180
(702) 876-5535

New Hampshire
Board of Registration in PT
Medicine
2 Industrial Park Dr.
Concord, NH 03301
(603) 271-1203

New Jersey
NJ State Board of PT
124 Halsey St., 6th Floor
P.O. Box 45014
Newark, NJ 07101
(201) 504-6455

New Mexico
NM Licensing Board
P.O. Box 25101
725 St. Michaels Dr.
Santa Fe, NM 87504
(505) 827-7162

New York
State Board for PT
Cultural Education Ctr.,
Room 3019
Albany, NY 12230
(518) 474-6374

North Carolina
NC Board of PT
Examiners
18 W. Colony Place, #120
Durham, NC 27705
(919) 490-6393

North Dakota
ND State Examining
Committee for PT
P.O. Box 69
Grafton, ND 58237
(701) 352-0125

Ohio
OH AT-PT Board
77 S. High St., 16th Floor
Columbus, OH 43266
(614) 466-3774

Oklahoma
OK State Board of
Med. License
P.O. Box 18256
5104 N. Francis, Suite C
Oklahoma City, OK 73154
(405) 848-6841

Oregon
OR PT Licensing Board
800 NE Oregon St.
Suite 407
Portland, OR 97232
(503) 731-4047

Pennsylvania
PA State Board of PT
P.O. Box 2649
Harrisburg, PA 17105
(717) 783-7134

Rhode Island
RI Dept. of Health-Div. of
Prof. Reg.
3 Capitol Hill,
104 Cannon Bldg.
Providence, RI 02908
(401) 277-2827

South Carolina
Dept. of Labor, Lic.,
and Regulations
3600 Forest Dr.
P.O. Box 11329
Columbia, SC 29211-1329
(803) 734-4170

South Dakota
SD Board of Medicine
1323 S. Minnesota Ave.
Sioux Falls, SD 57105
(605) 336-1965

Tennessee
TN Committee on PT
283 Plus Park Blvd.
Nashville, TN 37247
(615) ~~367-6225~~

Texas
TX State Board of PT
Examiners
3001 S. Lamar, Suite 101
Austin, TX 78704
(512) 443-8202

Utah
Div. of Occup. &
Prof. Licensing
160 E. 300 South
P.O. Box 45805
Salt Lake City, UT 84145
(801) 530-6767

Vermont
Office of Prof.
Reg.-Licensing & Regist.
109 State St.
Montpelier, VT 05609
(802) 828-2390

Virginia
Dept. of Health Prof.-VA
1601 Rolling Hills Dr.
Richmond, VA 23229
(804) 662-9924

Washington
Board of Med. Dept. of
Health
1300 SE Quince St.
P.O. Box 47868
Olympia, WA 98504-7868
(206) 753-3132

West Virginia
WV Board of PT
Rt. 1, Box 306
Creek, WV 26385
(304) 745-4161

Wisconsin
Dept. of Reg. &
Licensing-Med. Exam Lost
Brd.
P.O. Box 8935
Madison, WI 53708
(608) 267-9377

Wyoming
WY State Board of PT
2301 Central Ave.
Barrett Bldg.
3rd Floor
Cheyenne, WY 82002
(307) 777-7788

Chapter 2
The Job Search

Currently in the United States, there is a severe shortage of trained physical therapists and physical therapist assistants. There simply are not enough American therapists to meet the demands of the healthcare industry. Because of this, it will be extremely easy for you to find a job working in a facility in America. In fact, it is almost impossible **not** to find a job working as a PT or PTA. You will find that the institutions will be very helpful, usually assisting you with the licensing and visa procedures. You can expect to earn a salary anywhere from $35,000 to $80,000 or more per year, depending on the amount and type of experience you have, and the facility.

In addition to your salary, many facilities will pay you bonuses and relocation assistance. Because therapists are in such great demand, often a facility will pay you bonus money just to begin working there or give you money to cover the expense of moving to another location.

Facilities may be willing to give you additional money for working there if you are dealing directly with them and not using a recruiter. A **recruiter** is a person who acts as the connector between the therapist and the facility. For providing a therapist to a facility, the facility pays the recruiter a large fee (thousands of dollars). Dealing with the facility directly eliminates the recruiter and saves the facility a large sum of money.

We usually recommend trying to find a job without using a recruiter because of the reason we just mentioned, but also because often when you get a job offer through a recruiter you will have to sign a three or more year contract with the facility. Because the facility is paying thousands of dollars to the recruiter, they want to make certain that you will not leave anytime soon. It is better for you to have a one year (two at the most) contract, so that you can have a choice of where to work.

If you are overseas and you find the job search too difficult to do alone, however, using a recruiter isn't a bad idea. It is certainly the easiest way to find a job, and there are no direct costs to you–the hospital pays all of the fees.

In the remainder of this chapter, we will explain the different types of facilities available to you, the sources for finding these places, how to interview by phone and in person, and preparing your resumé.

Types of Facilities

The healthcare industry in the United States is large and rather complicated. There are many different types of treatment centers that specialize in different areas or operate a certain way. If you intend on working in the United States as a PT, you should know what these different types of facilities are and what they do.

Hospital: Treats all kinds of patients on an inpatient (sleeps overnight) and outpatient (patient leaves the same day-no overnight stay) basis. The same as a hospital in your country.

Nursing Home: A facility that treats mostly elderly patients.

Outpatient Clinic: Same day surgery and/or therapy. The patient does not spend the night in an outpatient clinic.

Home Health Care: A system that treats patients in their own homes. There are thousands of home health care agencies in America that work directly with patients who require treatment in their homes. As a therapist, this is one of the better-paying types of jobs.

School District: This type of job involves work with children in schools, either in special education (retardation, handicapped) or in sports education.

Sources for Your Job Search

The easiest way to find employers who are searching for therapists is to get a monthly publication that has pages and pages of facilities that are trying to hire PTs. If you are outside of the United States and you cannot find these journals in your library, call them directly and ask them to send the journals to you.

Physical Therapy Bulletin (703) 548-5482
Physical Therapy Forum (215) 337-0381

Another source for potential employers can be found by calling the board of physical therapy for the state you are interested in. They can send you a monthly bulletin of available jobs in that state.

Finally, if you are in the United States, you can go to a medical library and find a book called *The American Hospice Association Guide (AHA Guide)*. This book lists all of the hospitals in the United States. Also try the *Medical and Health Information Directory*.

Interviewing

Whether you are speaking on the telephone or in person, it is very important to make a good impression on a potential employer by having a successful interview. Basically, an interview is a way for both sides to find out about each other. It is a way for the employer to decide whether you would be right for the facility and it is a way for you to decide whether you would like to work there.

The first step is to call the facility and ask for the *human resources department* (if the telephone number is from an advertisement, it may be directly to the human resources department).

The second step is to tell the person: "I am calling to find out if you have any openings for a physical therapist." If you are answering an advertisement, you would say: "I am calling about the ad for a physical therapist." Be prepared for an interview.

The three most important things an employer is looking at in an interview are:

1. Your English skills: Can you communicate easily?
2. Your knowledge of physical therapy: Are you familiar with the latest treatments and techniques?
3. Your attitude and personality: Are you flexible? Can you adapt easily to new situations? Are you easy to work with? Are you friendly?

Here are some of the most common questions that the employer is likely to ask you:

- How long have you been working as a PT?
- What kind of experience do you have? (This means your previous work.)
- What kinds of patients have you worked with?
- What kinds of patients would you like to work with?
- Why do you want to come to the United States?
- Where did you go to school?
- How much money do you want to make? (You should answer: "I am open right now.")
- How big was the facility you worked in? (They may ask this question in terms of how many beds the facility had.)

While the interviewer is asking you questions, do not be afraid to ask questions of your own. In fact, ask as many *intelligent* questions as possible. We emphasize the word *intelligent* here because there is a difference between an intelligent and an ignorant question. Employers like to see that you are experienced and that you understand the field that you work in by being able to ask good questions. For example, a question such as "What is the difference between an outpatient and an inpatient clinic?" would *not* be a good one to ask on an interview. It shows your lack of knowledge of the industry. On the other hand, a question such as "Do you have an outpatient clinic?" shows that you understand the concepts and are selective in your job choice. Here are some other good questions to ask:

- How big is your hospital?
- How many patients a day do you treat?
- How many therapists do you have on staff?
- What kinds of patients do you treat?
- Would I be working on a rotation basis?(This means moving from one unit to another.)
- Do you provide any continuing education programs? (Sometimes the facility will pay for you to take additional courses in physical therapy.)
- What kind of benefits do you provide? (Medical, dental insurance)
- Do you offer any sign-up bonuses and relocation assistance?
- Do you take care of all of the necessary housing arrangements? (Usually the facility will arrange the housing, flight, airport pick-up, etc.)

Remember: you are trying to make a good impression on this person–sound as natural and friendly as possible. If you are going on a face-to-face interview (not on the telephone) dress very professionally in a suit. Shake hands firmly and look directly into the person's eyes when saying "Hello, nice to meet you." At the end of the interview, shake hands again and say "Thank you for your time." Also, remember to bring an extra copy of your resumé (explained below). Be confident without appearing arrogant.

Preparing Your Resumé

A resumé (sometimes called a CV) is a one or two page paper that summarizes your educational and professional work experience. Often, an employer will not even speak to you until they have your resume in their hands so they know who they are talking to. Sometimes when you see an advertisement for a job opening, it will simply say send resumé and cover letter to the following address. In this case, they want you to send your resumé along with a very short letter saying why you wish to have that particular job and why you are qualified. Sometimes you can call and talk to the human resources department for a while, and they will end the conversation by asking you to send a resumé.

The resumé is the formal representation of yourself. It should be as professional and neat as possible. We have provided a sample resumé for you to use to create your resumé. We recommend using the same type of layout.

Of course this sample resumé will be different to fit your own individual history. You may have additional educational credentials, more detailed work experience, or miscellaneous information that could be added, such as any publications you were involved in, or special skills that you may have. Remember, the resumé is a tool that is used to sell yourself–don't be afraid to write about **all** of the professional experience you have had. It is impossible to be boastful on a resumé.

First Name, Last Name
Address
City, State, Country
Phone

EDUCATION:

University of ???? - City, Country.
M.A. Physical Therapy (19??)

WORK EXPERIENCE:

??? Physical Therapy Company - City, Country.
(January 19?? - Present)
Working as a physical therapist in all areas of treatment, including cases in neurology, orthopedics, and acute care.

Orthopedic Clinic of ??? - City, Country
(November 19?? - October 19??)
Worked as a physical therapist concentrating on orthopedic cases. A significant amount of time working as a pediatric therapist in this clinic.

??? Hospital - City, Country
(May 19?? - October 19??)
Focused on cases involving neurological physical therapy. Also worked with acute care, geriatric and pediatric patients.

MISCELLANEOUS:

Fluent in English, French, Polish, German, ?

Chapter 3
Visas

A visa is a document that allows a foreign-born individual to enter or live in another country. There are many different types of visas available, depending on many different factors. For the purpose of a foreign-trained physical therapist, however, we can focus on two types of visa status:

Note to PTAs: You **cannot** come to the United States on a working visa as a PTA. If you are already in the United States, you can still get a temporary license in certain states and apply for a Green Card, but you can't work on a working visa.

Working Visa (H-1B): This is the visa that allows you to enter the United States for the purpose of legally earning money as a physical therapist (physical therapist assistants cannot come to the United States on a working visa as a PTA). The visa is valid for a period as long as the contract you sign with your sponsor (explained later). Note that this working visa is **only** valid for work as a physical therapist in the institution that hired you. You can't choose to legally do other jobs while on an H-1B visa.

Permanent Resident Status (Green Card): This is the ultimate goal for many foreign people who wish to live and work for long periods in the United States. Having a Green Card allows you to live and work anywhere you wish, for as long as you wish. You can travel freely between the United States and other countries without restrictions. Basically, you have the same rights as any American citizen, with the exception of being able to vote. Once you pass the national examination, it will be very easy for you to get your Green Card.

What Should I Do?

Basically, there are three situations that a foreign-trained therapist can face:

1. Being in your home (or a different) country and wanting to come to the U.S.
2. Being in the U.S. already on a visa
3. Being in the United States illegally.

Let's look carefully at each situation.

Coming from another country: In order to come to the United States to work as a physical therapist you must have a **sponsor**. In this case, a sponsor is simply a facility that is going to hire you as an employee. Once you have found a facility that you want to work in and that wants to hire you, the facility will do all of the necessary paperwork to get your visa. The facility will require your diploma and either your temporary license (if the state you will be working in issues temporary licenses) or credentials evaluation. The facility will provide an **offer of employment**, which is a formal document that verifies that they want to hire you. After all of the necessary documents are submitted, it will usually take 7 to 14 days to receive your working visa.

Already in the U.S. on a working visa: If you are in the United States on a working visa and you fail the exam, you can no longer legally work in America. As we explained in the previous chapter, however, you can still legally stay in the U.S. until the end of your working visa and try to pass the examination.

Already in the U.S. illegally: This is a situation which you do not want to be in, but if for some reason you are a foreign-trained physical therapist living illegally in the United States, there is hope for you.

The first thing you must do is find an employer who wants to hire you and be your sponsor. You can then choose to try to apply for a working visa or a Green Card. This is possible right now because the job of PT falls under a special law in the United States which allows foreign people to work here in jobs that are understaffed.

To get a working visa in this case you will have to first go back to your country to pick up the visa. This is a quick procedure–30 days maximum.

If you are going to try to get a Green Card, you can stay here while trying to adjust your status. You will have to pay money as a penalty and the waiting time could be as long as a year. Even though you may wait a long time for the Green Card, you can probably begin working in about four months or so. We recommend this option for people who have already been living in the U.S. for a long time, or for people who don't feel comfortable going back to their home country.

More About Green Cards

Once you have passed the national exam and have received your permanent license, it will be very easy for you to get your Green Card (for PTAs as well, but it may take a little more time). It is a good idea, however, to try to get your Green Card while you have your **temporary** license. In this way, even if you do not pass the exam, you can still continue living and working in the U.S. (as a rehab aide or any other job, but not as a PT) for as long as you want while you are preparing for the exam again.

The important thing to determine is how long your temporary license will be valid and what the Green Card situation is in the state you are in. Although the national laws are the same, each state is different regarding how long the wait is to receive your Permanent Resident Status, depending on how busy the office is at the time. In states such as Illinois, where there is a large immigrant population, it can take as long as a year to complete the entire process. In contrast, in a state such as Idaho it may take only 1 or 2 months to get your Green Card.

If your temporary license will expire before the estimated time of completing the application process (you can ask a state immigration office how long the wait is for a Green Card), do **not** apply for a Green Card. In this case, wait until you have a permanent license.

When applying for Permanent Residency, you might find the process easier if you hire an immigration lawyer to help you. Be aware, though, that this can be an expensive way to go. The **first** thing you should do is ask the facility you are involved with to help you with any immigration paperwork. If they are unwilling or unable to help you, and you do not want to complete the forms on your own (available at any immigration office), you can hire an attorney.

When choosing a lawyer, be sure to "shop around." Don't be afraid to ask as many questions as you like. Remember, a lawyer works for **you**. You pay them to work for you. If you don't feel comfortable with a particular lawyer, find another one. If there is one thing America has plenty of, it's lawyers. Be sure to find out exactly what the cost will be and how long you can expect to wait. Depending on where you are, the fee could be as high as $2000–but should be **no more** than this.

Chapter 4
Test Information

For **physical therapists**:

200 test questions
4 hours to complete the exam

Here is the breakdown of question types (issued by Professional Examination Service):

21% I. **Evaluation of the patient's/client's conditions**

A. Obtain patient history
B. Examine/assess musculoskeletal status
C. Examine/assess neuromuscular status
D. Examine/assess cardiopulmonary status
E. Examine/assess integumentary status
F. Examine/assess functional status
G. Examine/assess family and community support systems
H. Identify and interpret significant findings from evaluation

23% II. **Planning of the treatment program**

A. Short-term and long-term goals
B. Procedures, modalities, and equipment
C. Frequency of treatment
D. Delegation of appropriate parts of the treatment program
E. Consultation with and referral to other health care professionals

34% III. **Implementation of the treatment program**

A. Implement a therapeutic exercise program
B. Perform mobilization/manipulation techniques
C. Administer therapeutic modalities
D. Instruct in functional training
E. Prescribe, make, and/or apply assistive and adaptive devices
F. Implement a cardiopulmonary program
G. Perform skin care
H. Implement emergency care procedures
I. Instruct the patient/family support people
J. Assess treatment outcome and modify treatment plan/goals
K. Plan for discharge and continuity of care

11% IV. **Administration**

A. Communication and documentation
B. Implementation and monitoring of policies and procedures
C. Ethical and legal standards

9% V. **Education and consultation**

A. Planning and development of educational materials
B. Implementation and monitoring of educational materials

2% VI. **Research**

A. Read and interpret research data/literature
B. Evaluate and/or participate in research activities

For **physical therapist assistants**:

150 test questions
3 hours to complete exam

Here is the breakdown of question types (issued by Professional Examination Service):

32% I. **Examination of the patient/client**

- A. Observation and measurement of musculoskeletal status
- B. Observation and measurement of neuromuscular status
- C. Observation and measurement of cardiopulmonary status
- D. Observation and measurement of integumentary status
- E. Observation and measurement of functional status

57% II. **Implementation of the treatment program**

- A. Implement a therapeutic exercise program
- B. Administer therapeutic modalities
- C. Perform functional training
- D. Apply and measure assistive/adaptive devices
- E. Implement a cardiopulmonary treatment program
- F. Perform skin care
- G. Adhere to safety and emergency care procedures
- H. Identify changes in treatment outcome

11% III. **Communication, documentation, and ethical and legal standards**

- A. Communicate with supervising physical therapist
- B. Communicate with other health care professionals
- C. Communicate with patient and family
- D. Review medical records
- E. Document client/patient physical therapy care
- F. Participate in quality assurance programs
- G. Instruct patient and caregivers
- H. Use patient education materials
- I. Maintain ethical and legal standards
    1. Confidentiality
    2. Informed consent
    3. Documentation
    4. Professional responsibility

Chapter 5
Test-Taking Method

We suggest using this method while you are taking the practice exam and during the actual exam. It is okay to write on the questions, but not on the answer sheet.

1. Go to questions #50, #100 (and #150 for PT) and draw a line under the question with your pencil. This is a way of managing your time. When you get to a question with a line under it, you should check the time to be sure you are not far behind schedule.

2. Begin each item by reading the entire question (but not the four answer choices yet).

3. Underline the key words and phrases of the question. (This allows you to quickly understand what is important in the question without re-reading everything when you are looking at it again.)

4. Circle the pivotal words (*never, except, most, not,* etc.) of the question.

5. Try to think quickly of what the answer is **before** reading the choices.

6. Read **all** of the answer choices before choosing one.

7. If the answer you thought is correct is one of the choices, choose it. (Your first instinct is usually correct.)

8. If you are not immediately sure of which is the correct answer, eliminate the ones you know are **incorrect**.

9. When eliminating incorrect answers, put a line through the answer with your pencil.

10. If you are still not sure of the correct answer, make a guess based on any experience you may have.

11. If you have absolutely **no** idea which answer is correct, follow these rules for guessing:
    a. Choose the answer that looks most like all of the others
    b. Avoid answers that have very definite, strong language (i.e., *always, never,* etc.)
    c. Don't choose the same letter that would make a string of 3 in a row (i.e., #13 (C), #14(C), #15... you are guessing... don't guess (C).

Note: These "rules" should only be used as a very last chance effort. If you have any reason to think one answer is correct, choose it before using these guidelines.

12. Put a '?' next to the questions that you guessed at.

13. If you have time remaining after completing the exam, go back and look at the answers you put a '?' next to.

14. Make sure that you only spend 1 hour per 50 questions (approximately 1 1/4 minutes per question–maximum of 3 minutes per question).

15. Change an answer **only** if:
    Your first answer was a complete guess and after reading the item again you remember something you hadn't thought of before.
    You misread the question the first time (maybe you didn't notice *except*, for example).

Chapter 6
Highlighting Exercise

For these 20 questions, read each question completely and then use the technique of underlining the important words and circling the pivotal ones. Use the process of elimination when going through the answers. In Chapter 7, we have provided you with the same questions highlighted.

1. An obese 35-year-old woman with psoriasis has been referred to you for treatment. The disease has progressed throughout her upper extremities and she complains of itching. The most effective form of treatment for this patient would be:
A. ultrasound
B. whirlpool
C. ultraviolet radiation
D. none of the above treatments would be appropriate

2. There are many good reasons for keeping records about therapy treatment for each patient. The primary purpose for these records, however, is:
A. improving the quality of patient care
B. malpractice law suits
C. communication of patient care
D. improving the quality of care assessment

3. A 60-year-old female patient with lower back pain needs ultrasound treatment. During the treatment process, the patient begins to complain of a burning pain. Her reaction is an indication of:
A. too much medium
B. the sound head being moved too quickly
C. insufficient medium
D. none of the above

4. A 17-year-old patient sustains a closed head injury while horseback riding. Initially, the patient is awake and alert, however later he becomes drowsy and falls into a coma. You should suspect that the patient is suffering from a:
A. intracerebellar hematoma
B. intracerebral hematoma
C. acute subdural hematoma
D. subacute subdural hematoma

5. All of the following symptoms are characteristic of multiple sclerosis except:
A. muscle weakness
B. sensory disturbances
C. frequent convulsions
D. unilateral visual loss

6. As a home health care physical therapist, you receive a telephone call from your agency requesting that you allow a representative from Medicare to observe you while treating a patient. You call the patient to get permission for this visit, but the patient refuses. The most appropriate response would be to:
A. call your supervisor, because the patient has a right to refuse other visitors
B. explain to the patient that this is very important and he or she should reconsider
C. ignore the patient's refusal and bring the Medicare observer with you anyway
D. call the Medicare representative and explain the situation

7. While treating your 50-year-old male patient who has been diagnosed with Parkinson's disease, you notice that the patient cannot perform tapping movements quickly and smoothly. This condition is known as:
A. nystagmus
B. adiadochokinesis
C. reaction time
D. sialorrhea

8. A 65-year-old male patient has sustained a cerebrovascular accident. After an evaluation, you find that the patient has left-sided weakness of the upper and lower extremities. The affected area is likely to be found in the:
A. cerebellum
B. medulla
C. brainstem
D. right cerebral hemisphere

9. Embolism is least likely from:
A. thrombophlebitis
B. phlebothrombosis
C. deep thrombophlebitis
D. deep phlebothrombosis

10. A 5-year-old boy has suffered a fractured femur while playing in a tree. You should expect new bone formation to begin on the inner and outer surfaces of the damaged bone within:
A. 48 hours
B. 96 hours
C. 6 days
D. 9 days

11. You are a therapist working in an outpatient clinic. A woman comes in with her overweight teenage son who is complaining of moderate groin and knee pain. While you are testing the hip flexors, the leg abducts and externally rotates. The most likely diagnosis is:
A. Calve-Legg-Perthes disease
B. slipped capital femoral epiphysis
C. fracture of femoral head
D. sprained hip

12. As a pediatric therapist, you are treating an infant who has been diagnosed with acetabular dysplasia of the hip. During treatment, the baby begins to cry and scream and seems generally agitated. In this degree of congenital dysplasia, you should expect to find:
A. dislocation of the hip
B. that the acetabulum is shallow but the head of the femur remains seated
C. subluxation of the hip
D. all of the above

13. A therapist is doing an initial evaluation for a 32-year-old female patient with a partially torn anterior cruciate ligament of the right knee as a result of a skiing accident. The patient is unsure if she is supposed to continue wearing the splint given to her by her physician. The most appropriate course of action would be to:
A. tell the patient to wear the splint all the time
B. tell the patient not to use the splint because it would reduce muscle strength
C. tell the patient to use the brace only half of the day
D. none of the above

14. A 58-year-old female who lives with her husband and three children is a secretary. She has been referred to you for physical therapy after a stroke. During your initial evaluation, you found that although she has fair mobility, she is unable to talk or name common objects. This condition is best known as:
A. anomia
B. apraxia
C. receptive aphasia
D. agraphia

15. While walking home from your hospital one day, you meet an old friend who begins to tell you about her son who has been diagnosed with chronic brain syndrome. She asks you about your experience treating these types of patients. You tell her that all of the following conditions are commonly seen with this affliction except:

A. speech impairment
B. loss of memory
C. impairment in judgment
D. intellectual decline

16. Muscle atrophy is one of the complications that can occur as the result of a fracture. Volkman's ischemic contracture is another type of complication that can also occur. This condition can be found:

A. after a fracture of the neck
B. after a fracture in the upper extremities
C. as a result of a low arterial blood supply
D. as a result of an interference with the venous return

17. During your treatment of a 62-year-old car salesman, the patient suddenly complains of a sharp chest pain. You report the incident to the attending physician, who conducts several tests on the patient. The results of the tests show hemoptysis, tachycardia, and dyspnea. These symptoms probably indicate that the patient suffered a:

A. stroke
B. heart attack
C. pulmonary infarction
D. there is not enough information to make a proper diagnosis

18. You are a therapist working at a rehabilitation center and treat many patients over a long period of time. One patient, a 33-year-old banker, has been receiving therapy for a spinal cord injury sustained in a motor vehicle accident. The patient required a great deal of individual attention, so a closer than usual relationship naturally developed. At the end of treatment, the patient wants to show his gratitude to you by giving you a small amount of money. The appropriate response in this situation is to:

A. take the money, but be sure to tell your supervisor
B. take the money, but do not tell your supervisor
C. tell the patient that all extra money must be given to the director of the center so he or she can distribute it to all of the therapists
D. tell the patient that you cannot accept any money from patients

19. You are treating a patient who has suffered a cerebral vascular accident. During transfer training, the patients falls hard on the floor, but doesn't appear to be injured, as he gets up quickly by himself and sits in a nearby chair. Which of the following responses would be most appropriate?

A. continue treatment normally
B. call your supervisor immediately and fill out an accident report
C. call the patient's physician immediately
D. continue treatment and tell your supervisor about the incident when you are finished with treatment

20. You are treating a 45-year-male patient with an above knee amputation. While doing gait training, you notice that the patient is walking with a wide base of support. All of the following are possible causes of this gait deviation except:

A. short prosthesis
B. long prosthesis
C. abduction contracture
D. instability

Chapter 7
Key to Highlighting Exercise

Here is the best way to highlight the "core" of each question. Your highlighting may be slightly different, but should be very similar. The answers are also given for each question.

1. An obese 35-year-old woman with psoriasis has been referred to you for treatment. The disease has progressed throughout her upper extremities and she complains of itching. The most effective form of treatment for this patient would be:
A. ultrasound
B. whirlpool
C. ultraviolet radiation
D. none of the above treatments would be appropriate

2. There are many good reasons for keeping records about therapy treatment for each patient. The primary purpose for these records, however, is:
A. improving the quality of patient care
B. malpractice law suits
C. communication of patient care
D. improving the quality of care assessment

3. A 60-year-old female patient with lower back pain needs ultrasound treatment. During the treatment process, the patient begins to complain of a burning pain. Her reaction is an indication of:
A. too much medium
B. the sound head being moved too quickly
C. insufficient medium
D. none of the above

4. A 17-year-old patient sustains a closed head injury while horseback riding. Initially, the patient is awake and alert, however later he becomes drowsy and falls into a coma. You should suspect that the patient is suffering from a:
A. intracerebellar hematoma
B. intracerebral hematoma
C. acute subdural hematoma
D. subacute subdural hematoma

5. All of the following symptoms are characteristic of multiple sclerosis except:
A. muscle weakness
B. sensory disturbances
C. frequent convulsions
D. unilateral visual loss

6. As a home health care physical therapist, you receive a telephone call from your agency requesting that you allow a representative from Medicare to observe you while treating a patient. You call a patient to get permission for this visit, but the patient refuses. The most appropriate response would be to:
A. call your supervisor, because the patient has a right to refuse other visitors
B. explain to the patient that this is very important and he or she should reconsider
C. ignore the patient's refusal and bring the Medicare observer with you anyway
D. call the Medicare representative and explain the situation

7. While treating your 50-year-old male patient who has been diagnosed with Parkinson's disease, you notice that the patient cannot perform tapping movements quickly and smoothly. This condition is known as:
A. nystagmus
B. adiadochokinesis
C. reaction time
D. sialorrhea

8. A 65-year-old male patient has sustained a cerebrovascular accident. After an evaluation, you find that the patient has left-sided weakness of the upper and lower extremities. The affected area is likely to be found in the:
A. cerebellum
B. medulla
C. brainstem
D. right cerebral hemisphere

9. Embolism is least likely from:
A. thrombophlebitis
B. phlebothrombosis
C. deep thrombophlebitis
D. deep phlebothrombosis

10. A 5-year-old boy has suffered a fractured femur while playing in a tree. You should expect new bone formation to begin on the inner and outer surfaces of the damaged bone within:
A. 48 hours
B. 96 hours
C. 6 days
D. 9 days

11. You are a therapist working in an outpatient clinic. A woman comes in with her overweight teenage son who is complaining of moderate groin and knee pain. While you are testing the hip flexors, the leg abducts and externally rotates. The most likely diagnosis is:
A. Calve-Legg-Perthes disease
B. slipped capital femoral epiphysis
C. fracture of femoral head
D. sprained hip

12. As a pediatric therapist, you are treating an infant who has been diagnosed with acetabular dysplasia of the hip. During treatment, the baby begins to cry and scream and seems generally agitated. In this degree of congenital dysplasia, you should expect to find:
A. dislocation of the hip
B. that the acetabulum is shallow but the head of the femur remains seated
C. subluxation of the hip
D. all of the above

13. A therapist is doing an initial evaluation for a 32-year-old female patient with a partially torn anterior cruciate ligament of the right knee as a result of a skiing accident. The patient is unsure if she is supposed to continue wearing the splint given to her by her physician. The most appropriate course of action would be to:
A. tell the patient to wear the splint all the time
B. tell the patient not to use the splint because it would reduce muscle strength
C. tell the patient to use the brace only half of the day
D. none of the above

14. A 58-year-old female who lives with her husband and three children is a secretary. She has been referred to you for physical therapy after a stroke. During your initial evaluation, you found that although she has fair mobility, she is unable to talk or name common objects. This condition is best known as:
A. anomia
B. apraxia
C. receptive aphasia
D. agraphia

15. While walking home from your hospital one day, you meet an old friend who begins to tell you about her son who has been diagnosed with chronic brain syndrome. She asks you about your experience treating these types of patients. You tell her that all of the following conditions are commonly seen with this affliction except:

A. speech impairment
B. loss of memory
C. impairment in judgment
D. intellectual decline

16. Muscle atrophy is one of the complications that can occur as the result of a fracture. Volkman's ischemic contracture is another type of complication that can also occur. This condition can be found:

A. after a fracture of the neck
B. after a fracture in the upper extremities
C. as a result of a low arterial blood supply
D. as a result of an interference with the venous return

17. During your treatment of a 62-year-old car salesman, the patient suddenly complains of a sharp chest pain. You report the incident to the attending physician, who conducts several tests on the patient. The results of the tests show hemoptysis, tachycardia, and dyspnea. These symptoms probably indicate that the patient suffered a:

A. stroke
B. heart attack
C. pulmonary infarction
D. there is not enough information to make a proper diagnosis

18. You are a therapist working at a rehabilitation center and treat many patients over a long period of time. One patient, a 33-year-old banker, has been receiving therapy for a spinal cord injury sustained in a motor vehicle accident. The patient required a great deal of individual attention, so a closer than usual relationship naturally developed. At the end of treatment, the patient wants to show his gratitude to you by giving you a small amount of money. The appropriate response in this situation is to:

A. take the money, but be sure to tell your supervisor
B. take the money, but do not tell your supervisor
C. tell the patient that all extra money must be given to the director of the center so he or she can distribute it to all of the therapists
D. tell the patient that you cannot accept any money from patients

19. You are treating a patient who has suffered a cerebral vascular accident. During transfer training, the patients falls hard on the floor, but doesn't appear to be injured, as he gets up quickly by himself and sits in a nearby chair. Which of the following responses would be most appropriate?

A. continue treatment normally
B. call your supervisor immediately and fill out an accident report
C. call the patient's physician immediately
D. continue treatment and tell your supervisor about the incident when you are finished with treatment

20. You are treating a 45-year-old male patient with an above knee amputation. While doing gait training, you notice that the patient is walking with a wide base of support. All of the following are possible causes of this gait deviation except:

A. short prosthesis
B. long prosthesis
C. abduction contracture
D. instability

Chapter 8
Multiple Choice Phrases

The multiple choice PT/PTA state licensing exams use some tricky phrases. Practice these phrases until you feel comfortable when you see them.

Here are the most common ones:

Which of the following ... (not) (isn't)
All of the following.... except
Which of the following... would you (not) expect to (find) (see) ...
The most appropriate (response) (action) ....
Which of the following would be inappropriate...
Which of the following statements...
All of the above
None of the above
Both (b) and (c)

1. Which of the following methods is an effective way of treating sore muscles?
   A. hot packs
   B. hot needles
   C. hot potatoes
   D. hot irons

2. Which of the following methods is *not* an effective way of treating sore muscles?
   A. hot packs
   B. cold packs
   C. exercise
   D. massage

3. All of the following methods are acceptable ways of treating sore muscles except:
   A. hot packs
   B. cold packs
   C. exercise
   D. massage

Note: If the phrase *all of the following* is used, the word *except* must always follow.

4. Which of the following methods would you expect to see being used to treat sore muscles?
   A. surgery
   B. x-rays
   C. cold packs
   D. hypnosis

5. A patient complains of sore muscles after playing basketball. The most appropriate response is to:
   A. tell the patient not to complain so much
   B. tell the patient to do proper stretching before playing and apply hot packs after.
   C. tell the patient not to play basketball anymore
   D. tell the patient to make an appointment with a physician

6. Which of the following treatments would be inappropriate for sore muscles?
   A. hot packs
   B. cold packs
   C. massage
   D. x-rays

7. Which of the following statements is true?
   A. hot packs are an effective way to treat sore muscles
   B. cold packs cause sore muscles
   C. hot packs can only be prescribed by a physician
   D. cold packs are an ineffective way of treating sore muscles

8. Which of the following methods are effective in treating sore muscles?
   A. hot packs
   B. cold packs
   C. massage
   D. all of the above are effective treatment methods.

Note: When you see *all of the above*, you only need to be **somewhat** sure that **two** of the answers are correct.

9. All of the following treatment methods are effective when treating sore muscles except:
   A. hot packs
   B. cold packs
   C. massage
   D. none of the above

Note: When you see *none of the above*, you only need to be **somewhat** sure that **none** of the answers are correct.

10. Which of the following methods are used to treat sore muscles?
    A. hypnosis
    B. hot packs
    C. cold packs
    D. both B and C

11. All of the following actions are considered reflexes except:
    A. sneezing
    B. laughing
    C. coughing
    D. blinking

12. Which of the following conditions would you *not* expect to see in a person immediately after surgery?
    A. strength
    B. pain
    C. swelling
    D. weakness

13. Which of the following statements is *not* an accurate description of an HMO?
    A. HMOs do not limit the amount of treatment time
    B. HMOs lower the cost to the patient
    C. HMOs do not cover the cost of medication
    D. all of the above are accurate descriptions of an HMO

14. The most appropriate response to an 11-year-old boy who does not want to listen while you are explaining a home program is to:
    A. ask a family member to come into the room while you are explaining the instructions
    B. tell the boy you will not help him because he is not listening
    C. continue with your instructions
    D. call your supervisor

15. Which of the following tasks would be inappropriate for a physical therapist assistant to perform?
    A. apply and measure assistive or adaptive devices
    B. identify changes in the outcome of treatment
    C. administer therapeutic modalities
    D. change a treatment plan or goals

16. A good way to avoid a lawsuit is to:
   A. keep accurate and timely records
   B. follow good ethical procedures
   C. increase malpractice insurance
   D. both A and B

17. Which of the following is considered an important stage of treatment?
   A. evaluation
   B. planning
   C. implementation
   D. all of the above

18. Which of the following terms would be used to describe a test that measures what it is supposed to measure?
   A. reliable
   B. significant
   C. valid
   D. experimental

19. A patient appears to have difficulty breathing, begins sweating profusely, and is holding his chest. The most appropriate action to would be to:
   A. do nothing and see if the patient begins to feel better
   B. call a physician immediately
   C. record the event in the patient's chart
   D. leave the room and give the patient some privacy

20. If you are not happy with the patient load you have because you think it is too difficult, an appropriate action would be to:
   A. talk directly to your supervising therapist about your feelings
   B. talk to other staff members and complain to them about your situation
   C. talk to the board of directors and explain the problem
   D. do nothing and try to work a little harder

21. You are testing the muscle strength of the ankle plantarflexors of a patient who has sustained a fracture of the talus. All of the following muscles provide plantarflexion for the ankle except:
   A. gastrocnemius
   B. tibialis anterior
   C. soleus
   D. peroneus longus

22. During isometric exercises, you can expect to find all of the following occurrences except:
   A. muscle contracting without a change in length
   B. no visible joint motion
   C. strength developing at position in which exercise is performed
   D. muscle contracting with change in the length

23. Which of the following is not a typical soft tissue lesion?
   A. sprain
   B. fracture
   C. strain
   D. subluxation

24. You are treating a patient with an acute tendon rupture of the shoulder. During the acute stage, it is normal to observe that there is pain and limited movement in the affected area. Which of the following are possible causes of this problem?

A. edema
B. muscle spasm
C. irritating chemicals
D. all of the above

25. While you are treating a patient who has sustained a fracture of the tibia, during the immobilization period you should expect to find all of the following except:

A. muscle atrophy
B. increased circulation
C. contracture formation
D. decreased circulation

26. Which of the following muscles causes compression and downward translation of the humerus?

A. infraspinatus
B. teres minor
C. subscapularis
D. all of the above

27. All of the following are valid uses of a SOAP note except:

A. research
B. quality assurance
C. scheduling
D. communication

28. All of the following are typical symptoms for myasthenia gravis except:

A. limb weakness
B. dysarthria
C. dysphasia
D. hemiplegia

29. You are treating a patient with a lesion of the inferior gluteal nerve. Which of the following motions would be the most affected?

A. hip extension
B. hip adduction
C. hip abduction
D. hip flexion

30. Which of the following are typical treatment goals for the acute stage of bursitis?

A. control of the amount of pain
B. control edema
C. maintain soft tissue and joint mobility
D. all of the above

Chapter 9
Prefixes and Suffixes

By knowing a list of common prefixes and suffixes, you will be able to better understand unfamiliar words, allowing you to understand the question correctly.

Suffixes

General:

-able: can do or can be
-ful: full or filled with
-less: without
-ly: the way something is (adverb)

Noun Suffixes:

-ion -sion -tion: All noun suffixes change words into nouns meaning
-ment either "the state of being" or "the act of doing."
-ity
-ness

Verb Suffixes:

-ify: These four verb suffixes indicate that a word is a verb meaning
-ate "to make," "to have," or "to become."
-en
-ize

-ing: an action in progress
-ed: past action

Adjective Suffixes:

-y: Adjective suffixes change words into adjectives meaning
-ous "like" or "related to."
-ish
-ic
-ive

Note: A prefix or suffix that is often used on the licensing exam is in **bold** and should be studied very carefully.

Prefixes

General:

re-: to do again
sub-: under, below, less than
co-: with, together
counter- (contra-): against, opposite

Negative Prefixes:

il-: not
im-: not
in-: not
ir-: not
un-: not

non-: not, without
a- (an-): without, lacking
anti-: against, opposite, preventing
dis-: not or remove
mal-: bad, poorly
mis-: wrongly, incorrectly

Position Prefixes:

ante-: before in time or place
pre-: before in time or place
post-: after in time or place
inter-: between in time or place
intra-: within

Movement Prefixes:

trans-: motion across something, or from place to place
de-: movement down, away from, or to remove or take off

Complete the following exercises using the chart of prefixes and suffixes. On the first line, write the root of the word in bold. On the second line, write the definition of the word with the suffix or prefix. Remember, some of the words may have both a prefix **and** a suffix.

---

1. During the operation, the doctor instructed the patient to remain **motionless.**

root:_______________

motionless:____

2. Although the patient was feeling better, the symptoms began to **reappear**.

root:_______________

reappear:____

3. To avoid **malpractice** lawsuits, doctors must be careful to diagnose the patient correctly.

root:_______________

malpractice:____

4. If a patient is having difficulty breathing, it is a good idea to remove all **restrictive** clothing.

root:_______________

restrictive:____

5. The new therapist **inaccurately** assessed the patient's problem.

root:_______________

inaccurately:____

6. Sometimes a therapist must apply **counterpressure** to a part of a patient's body.

root:_______________

counterpressure:____

7. If a patient seems unsure of what to expect during therapy, the therapist should explain the procedure before they **initiate** treatment.

root:_______________

initiate:____

8. When finding out a patient's history, you should not spend much time asking **irrelevant** questions.

root:_______________

irrelevant:____

9. Some of the newer casts that are made today are **immersible** in water.

root:_______________

immersible:____

10. When **instructing** patients on home care, it is important to make sure that they understand your directions clearly.

root:_______________

instructing:____

11. Aspirin is effective in the **reduction** of fever.

root:_______________

reduction:____

12. Sometimes you may not be sure of the best course of action. In these cases, you must use your best **judgment**.

root:_______________

judgment:____

13. You may need more patience when treating a **pre-adolescent** patient.

root:_______________

pre-adolescent:____

14. A child can usually sit **unsupported** at about 7 months of age.

root:_______________

unsupported:____

15. To **minimize** errors, a therapist should always pay close attention while filling out paperwork.

root:_______________

minimize:____

16. Many people in America have become **distrustful** of the health care system in this country.

root:_______________

distrustful:____

17. It is always important to have **objectivity** when evaluating a patient.

root:_______________

objectivity:____

18. One effective treatment for osteoarthritis is the use of **anti-inflammatory** drugs.

root:_______________

anti-inflammatory:____

19. **Improperly** wrapping an ankle could cause a problem with the patient's circulation.

root:_______________

improperly:____

20. **Weakness** of the immune system is what causes the eventual death of AIDS patients.

root:_______________

weakness:____

21. It is **atypical** for a woman to gain most of her weight during the second month of pregnancy.

root:_______________

atypical:____

22. Sometimes it takes a few hours for a person's ears to **depressurize** after flying in an airplane.

root:_______________

depressurize:____

23. A high fever can be dangerous, but an excessively **sub-normal** temperature can also cause problems for a patient.

root:_______________

sub-normal:____

24. A high **inter-tester** reliability means that two therapists who administer the same test to the same patient achieve similar results.

root:_______________

inter-tester:____

25. A high **intra-tester** reliability means that one therapist who administers the same test to the same patient two or more times achieves similar results each time.

root:_______________

intra-tester:____

26. If you write your notes **illegibly**, it will be difficult to read them.

root:_______________

illegibly:____

27. **Postoperative** pain is normal in many procedures.

root:_______________

postoperative:____

28. Because the doctor **misdiagnosed** the patient's problem, a lawsuit was pending against him.

root:_______________

misdiagnosed:____

29. Many insurance policies will not cover **nonessential** treatment procedures.

root:_______________

nonessential:____

30. **Therapeutic** exercises help the patient to regain their strength and energy.

root:_______________

therapeutic:____

Chapter 10
English Words

For each sentence, choose one word which **best** fits the entire meaning. Some sentences have more than one word which could be used, but since each word is only used once, you must select the word that works best for the whole sheet.

Note: Any word in bold is used in another exercise.

to assess (assessment)	to diagnose (diagnosis)	to evaluate (evaluation)
to measure (measurement)	to note	objectivity
to determine	criteria	to find (findings)
to identify	goals	results
to screen (screening)		

1. To _______________ what the best **treatment** for a patient will be, the therapist must do a complete and thorough **assessment**.

2. Therapists use many tests to _______________ the **amount** of **impairment** a patient has.

3. Only a doctor can make a(n) _______________ of a patient's problem.

4. To insure _______________ **during** an **evaluation**, a therapist should never ask a patient questions that imply a "correct" answer.

5. A physical therapist _______________ patients **in order to** define their specific needs.

6. Whether or not a patient still has **pain** is a good _______________ for **measuring** his or her **progress**.

7. Early _______________ can often detect diseases such as cancer, enabling successful **treatment**.

8. Often an x-ray cannot _______________ exactly what the problem is.

9. **Long-term** _______________ for a patient are always included in an **initial assessment**.

10. If you _______________ that a patient is having a difficult time breathing, you must quickly help him.

11. Recent _______________ have shown that smoking does cause cancer.

12. When the _______________ of a test are positive, some kind of **treatment** is **necessary**.

to appear (seem)	characteristic	to demonstrate (demonstration)
to exhibit	symptom	history of
sign	condition	to denote
background	to behave (behavior)	

1. One of the _______________ of influenza is fever.

2. If a patient begins to _______________ **signs** of a seizure, you must protect him from hurting himself.

3. The _______________ of a patient should be studied **before** a **treatment** plan is made.

4. Cerebral Palsy is a very **severe** _______________ which **affects** the brain and nervous system.

5. A patient who has a(an) _______________ heart problem in the family should regularly check his or her blood pressure.

6. Sometimes a patient's _______________ can become violent. In these cases, the therapist should **immediately** call for help.

7. One of the _______________ of HIV positive is a **chronic cough** and cold.

8. A patient _______________ to have injured her spinal cord. You are not sure, however, so further tests must be done.

9. A _______________ of Down's syndrome is mental retardation.

10. **In order to** make certain that a patient is **able** to do exercises at home, the therapist must first _______________ how to do them for the patient.

11. One of the many abbreviations used by physical therapists is **ROM**, which _______________ **range of motion**.

amount	excessive	normal	partial	fully	entire
majority	sufficient	total	more	most	decrease
increase	additional	certain	maximum (maximal)	minimum (minimal)	

1. If a patient has **burns** over 100% of his body, then we could say that his _______________ body has been **burned.**

2. If a patient has **burns** over 55% of his body, then we could say that the _______________ of his body has been **burned.**

3. It is _______________ difficult to **treat** a patient who is not cooperative than one who is.

4. _______________ inspiration is the **most** air a person can breathe into her lungs.

5. _______________ medical costs have made health insurance in America very expensive.

6. **In order to** be **effective**, a therapist must spend a(an) _______________ **amount** of time with each patient.

7. If a person **seems** to be choking but can still **cough**, this person has a(an) _______________ obstructed airway.

8. On the other hand, if a person is choking and cannot make any sound, this person has a(n) _______________ obstructed airway.

9. Therapists **conduct** exercise tests to **determine** the _______________ of **impairment.**

10. One of the **goals** of physical therapy is to _______________ **pain.**

11. Drinking a(n) _______________ **amount** of alcohol can lead to problems with your liver.

12. A physical therapy aide must be a(an) _______________ of 18 years old.

13. If you are not sure about how to **treat** a patient, you should get _______________ information from a supervisor.

14. There are usually many different types of exercises that can be done with a patient. It is the therapist's responsibility to **determine** the _______________ **appropriate** one.

15. _______________ injuries require **more treatment** than others.

16. Five weeks **after** the **accident**, the patient **discontinued** therapy because her **range of motion** was _______________.

17. The audit showed that a(n) _______________ of 40 hours of **treatment** had been given to the patient.

duration
short-term
frequency

immediate
long-term
occasionally

prolong
consistently

1. The ______________of one **treatment** session is usually 30-45 minutes long.

2. When a patient **sustains** a **deep laceration**, the ______________ response of the therapist should be to **apply** direct **pressure**.

3. Because the patient was still experiencing **pain**, the doctor decided to ______________ the **treatment**.

4. A(n) ______________ **benefit** is something that is good now but may or may not be good in the future.

5. A(n) ______________ **benefit** is something that may or may not be good now but is good in the future.

6. A therapist who is ______________ late for work will probably lose his job.

7. The number of times a patient receives **treatment** per week is called the ______________.

8. ______________ there will be a question about a patient's **treatment record.** In these cases, it is helpful if you have maintained **accurate notes**.

moderate	mild	severe
acute	chronic	

1. Of **moderate, mild,** and **severe pain**, the one that describes the **most** serious **condition** is _______________.

2. The least **amount** of **pain** of the descriptions above would be _______________.

3. So, we can say that _______________ **pain** would be a degree of **pain** somewhere in **between** _______________ and _______________.

4. A(n) _______________ **condition** is one that **continues** for a long time, usually years.

5. _______________ care patients have usually had surgery recently.

elevate	immerse	kneel	lower
raise	movable (immovable)	motion	rhythm
repetition	reflex	descend	ascend
ROM (range of motion)			

1. Very often, elderly people will have difficulty ______________ stairs without **assistance** because their muscles are not **strong** enough.

2. When ______________ stairs without **assistance**, elderly people must be careful not to slip and fall.

3. A regular, **normal** heartbeat has a steady ______________.

4. If you recently had surgery on your knees, it would be very **painful** to ______________.

5. A(n) ______________ is a body **motion** that we cannot control.

6. Minor **burns** should be **treated immediately** by ______________ the **affected** area in cool water.

7. If a person cannot rotate her shoulder **fully**, then we say that she has a limited ______________.

8. The therapist should **instruct** the patient to keep his foot ______________**after** spraining his ankle.

9. If a patient can move her arm, then her arm is ______________, but if she cannot move their arm it is ______________.

10. When adjusting the difficulty of a patient's exercises, the therapist can **either** increase the **amount** of resistance or the number of ______________.

11. The ______________ **extremities** are the legs.

12. The patient complained that his arm hurt only when he made one particular ______________.

13. A patient who cannot ______________ his arms above his head has a limited range of motion in his shoulders.

further	prior to	before
after	during	between
behind	position	initial

1. _______________ **performing** tests on a patient, a therapist must **record** the **results**.

2. A(n) _______________ **evaluation** is the first time the therapist **evaluates** a patient.

3. _______________ someone can become a physical therapist in America, she must pass the state licensing examination.

4. Sometimes a therapist may recommend that a patient sleep with a pillow _______________ his legs.

5. _______________ **treatment**, you should always be very attentive to the patient.

6. Because the **results** of the test were inconclusive, _______________ tests had to be done.

7. If you are **consistently** _______________ on your paperwork because your patient load is too heavy, you should tell the supervising physical therapist what the problem is.

8. A therapist must **record** the **vital signs** of a patient _______________ beginning physical therapy.

9. There are times when you must **treat** a patient in the supine _______________.

stretching	resistance	pressure	to place (placement)
technique	task	training	treatment
method	apply	touch	tension
stabilize	implement	stationary	

1. There are many different kinds of breathing _______________ to **treat** people with pulmonary problems.

2. The three stages of **treatment** are: **evaluate**, plan, and _______________.

3. The five senses of a human being are sight, hearing, smell, taste, and _______________.

4. When assisting elderly people to climb the stairs, you must instruct them to _______________ their hand firmly on the handrail for support and safety.

5. Gravity is something that provides natural _______________ when doing exercises.

6. A good therapist designs a(an) _______________ plan that will provide the **most benefit** to the patient.

7. If you see that a patient cannot do what you have asked him to do, it could be that the _______________ is too difficult.

8. You can recommend wrapping an ankle **during** activity to _______________ the **weak** joint.

9. Something that is _______________ does not move.

10. Depending on the situation, there are many different _______________ for **measuring** a patient's pulse.

11. A patient who has recently suffered a stroke may require gait _______________.

12. **Applying immediate** _______________ to a **laceration** is the best way to try to stop the bleeding.

13. One **method** for reducing **pain** is to _______________ hot packs.

14. **Before** an athlete begins playing her sport, she should always do _______________ exercises to loosen her muscles.

15. Massage is an **effective technique** for reducing muscle _______________.

swelling	burn	fracture	accident
deep laceration	cough	strain	sprain
rupture	weakness	pain	

1. A(n) _______________ is when a bone in the body is broken.

2. A muscle _______________ is often caused by overuse of a particular muscle.

3. A(n) _______________ is a **reflex** that can help to clear the throat.

4. _______________ are usually caused by fire or intense heat.

5. A common form of _______________ is a headache.

6. Ankles are often _______________ while playing sports. This is less **severe** than a **fracture**, which is an actual bone break.

7. _______________ actually **increases** the size of the **affected** area.

8. _______________ are harmful or negative events that are not done on purpose.

9. A(n) _______________ is when an internal organ breaks open.

10. A(n) _______________ is a very **severe** break in the skin that normally **results in** bleeding.

11. _______________ is an absence of **strength**.

complication	deviation	harmful	impairment
obese	tenderness	tight	unconscious
sustained injury	shortness of breath		

1. If a person becomes _______________ due to a head injury, there is a good chance the person has suffered a concussion.

2. There are times when a patient is **treated** successfully for his problem but is still sick due to _______________.

3. CVA patients will often suffer from speech _______________.

4. A patient with emphysema will probably experience _______________ when **ascending** stairs.

5. If a drug is found to be _______________, it is **immediately** removed from use.

6. A person who _______________ to her spinal cord is in danger of becoming paralyzed.

7. Insect bites often cause _______________ and **swelling** at the location of the bite.

8. When wrapping an ankle **sprain**, it is important not to make the bandage too _______________ so as to cut off blood circulation.

9. Anything that is not a **normal behavior** or test **result** is considered a(n) _______________.

10. Long ago, it was thought that _______________ people just ate too much. We now know that many times this problem is caused by a chemical imbalance.

to enter (entry)
to document (documentation)
to record (record)
discharge
HMO
inpatient
outpatient
litigation

1. _______________ have been one way to try to stop the **increasing** medical costs in the United States.

2. A patient is _______________ when a therapist **determines** that therapy is no longer **necessary**.

3. Maintaining **accurate records** is a good way to avoid _______________.

4. If a patient checks into the hospital as a(n) _______________, he will spend at least one night in the hospital.

5. When making _______________ in a patient's **record**, it is important to write neatly and clearly.

6. _______________ the **progress** of a patient is important for insurance purposes.

7. A(n) _______________ , on the other hand, leaves the hospital the same day of the medical procedure.

8. If a patient falls and injures herself **during treatment**, you must be sure to _______________ everything about the **accident**.

acceptable	necessary	essential	appropriate
accurate	effective	practical	viable
able			

1. In the past 10 or 15 years, acupuncture in America has become a(an) ______________ form of medical **treatment**.

2. It is not ______________ for a therapist to ask personal questions not related to **treatment**.

3. For a test to be ______________, it is **essential** that the therapist administer the test the same way each time.

4. Therapy tests are used to **determine** whether or not therapy is ______________.

5. Sometimes physical therapy is a(n) ______________ alternative to surgery.

6. If a patient is **obese**, you may not be ______________ to help move him out of bed.

7. Sometimes one **treatment method** would be more **effective** than another, but you can't use it because it is not ______________.

8. To obtain **valid** data on a test, it is ______________ that the therapist be **consistent** in her **methods**.

9. Radiation **treatment** has been proven to be ______________ in fighting cancer.

course of action
in order to
in and above

results in
associated with

allows for
out of proportion

1. A patient must _______________ a wound to heal **before** resuming his **normal** activities.

2. A patient with a(n) _______________ knee amputation has had his leg amputated above the knee.

3. At times there will be many choices to make. It will be up to the therapist to **determine** the best _______________

4. Lung cancer and emphysema are diseases _______________ cigarette smoking.

5. If a patient is **exhibiting behavior** that is _______________ to your **clinical results**, there may be some other factor causing this.

6. Lack of exercise _______________ a loss of muscle tone.

7. _______________ design a **proper** cardiac rehabilitation program, you must first understand the patient's **history**.

clinical significant validity reliability
statistical significance

1. _______________ is a term used to **determine** whether or not **results** of an experiment or test are due to chance.

2. A(n) _______________ **amount** of a therapist's time is spent **documenting treatment progress.**

3. If a test is _______________, this means that it will give **consistent results** each time it is given.

4. If a test is _______________, this means that it **measures** what it is supposed to **measure.**

5. A(n) _______________ **finding** is information that is obtained through **objective** tests.

variety
to review
to improve (improvement)
vary/varying
modify

1. A therapist can _______________ the settings of some modalities to be **appropriate** for each individual patient.

2. The main **goal** of physical therapy is to _______________ the overall quality of life of a patient.

3. Parkinson's disease has a(an) _______________ of **symptoms** including tremors, slow speech, and rigidity.

4. If you decide to **modify** a patient's **treatment**, it is a good idea to _______________ her chart and history.

5. If it **appears** as though **treatment** is not **effective** for a patient, then the **treatment** plan should be _______________.

to instruct (instruction)	to discuss (discussion)	to assist (assistance)
to obtain	to perform (performance)	to elicit
to continue	to attempt	to prevent (prevention)
to dismiss		

1. To _______________ injury, elderly people should be very careful when using the stairs.

2. Walkers are designed to _______________ patients who have a difficult time with their gait.

3. One way to _______________ relevant and **accurate** answers while **obtaining** a patient's history is to ask **objective** questions that do not lead the patient.

4. Along with **treating** the patient, it is the therapist's responsibility to _______________ the situation and **treatment** plan with the patient's family.

5. If a test **result** is not **statistically significant**, you must _______________ the information as chance.

6. When _______________ **strengthening** exercises, it is important not to add too much **resistance** so as to injure the patient.

7. If a patient must do exercises at home, it is important to _______________ him on how to do the exercises **properly**.

8. If a patient has not reached an **appropriate** level of functioning, physical therapy might have to be _______________.

9. You should always _______________ to give your patient the best possible **treatment** you can.

10. To _______________ a license to practice physical therapy in America, you must first pass a state licensing examination.

to provide	to utilize	to emphasize (emphasis)
to elect	to integrate	to delay
to apply (application)	compensate for	to conduct

1. After _______________ many tests, you find that the patient doesn't **appear** to have any physical problems. External consequences may be causing the problem.

2. Many managers in American hospitals have a strong _______________ on communication.

3. A person may **continue** to _______________ starting **treatment** because she is afraid of all medical procedures.

4. If a therapist does not like a hospital environment, he may _______________ to work as a home health care therapist.

5. A person tends to _______________ a weak or injured hand by using the good hand much more often.

6. A good therapist is **able** to _______________ good personal relationships with the patient along with **effective treatment**.

7. The management of the physical therapy department should _______________ each therapist with a manual containing all policies and procedures.

8. **Immediately after spraining** your ankle, the best **treatment** is to _______________ ice packs to the ankle.

9. Because there are so many patients in a day to be seen, a therapist must _______________ her time well.

to sense	to assume (assumption)	to expect (expectation)
to detect	consider	to comprehend
unknown		

1. **Applying** hot packs to back pain is _______________ an **effective treatment method**.

2. If you _______________ something unusual about a patient's breathing, you should watch her carefully to make sure she is okay.

3. You should _______________ to **find** swelling **immediately** following an operation.

4. A cure for AIDS is _______________ at this time.

5. You must be sure that a patient _______________ your instructions for care in the home.

6. The patient does not say so, but you can _______________ that he is unsure of what to **expect during** a massage of an injured muscle.

7. When doing an **initial evaluation**, it is important not to _______________ anything about a patient's **condition**.

to restrict (restriction)	to eliminate (elimination)	to disregard
to disrupt (disruption)	to diminish	to inhibit
failure to		

1. If a wound is not kept clean, the body's natural healing process will be _______________.

2. A therapist should never _______________ any orders given by a physician.

3. Anytime the blood supply is _______________, there is **potential** danger.

4. _______________ maintain accurate written records could **increase** the chance of legal problems.

5. The reason for a hard plaster cast for a broken bone is to _______________ the movement of the injured area.

6. A person's physical **strength** will naturally _______________ with age.

7. On a multiple choice exam, _______________ answers that you know are incorrect will help you **determine** which answer is correct.

benefit progress to facilitate support

1. One of the biggest ______________ of using a **Health Maintenance Organization** is the **decreased** cost to the patient.

2. To ______________ recovery, a patient must follow all of the orders the doctor and therapist prescribe.

3. Patients that have lower back problems should always make sure that they have adequate ______________.

4. A very satisfying part of being a therapist is watching the ______________ of a patient they are working with.

modality	to drain (drainage)	to secrete (secretion)
(pre)post-operative	intervention	3 weeks status post _____
precaution	ipsilateral	vital signs
extremities	internal	external
digits	contraindication	

1. If we say a patient is ______________ abdominal surgery, this means she had abdominal surgery 3 weeks ago.

2. The pituitary gland is responsible for ______________ a hormone that controls the body's metabolism.

3. One of the ______________ of heat therapy is sensory loss.

4. **During** surgery, patients' ______________ are continuously monitored to be sure they are in no danger.

5. Early ______________ can help to stop the spread of some diseases, such as cancer.

6. At times, a doctor may have to ______________ an infection before healing can begin.

7. A normal human body has 20 ______________ (10 toes and 10 fingers).

8. Many stroke patients have ______________ **impairment** so they can only use one arm.

9. Even though the person was not bleeding, he was hurt very badly because of ______________ injuries.

10. Normal ______________ reactions are **pain**, **swelling**, and **irritation**.

11. Hot packs are indicated for pain or muscle spasms, but ______________ for open wounds.

12. The upper ______________ are the arms, while the lower ______________ are the legs.

13. Some examples of therapeutic ______________ are: hot packs, ultrasound, and TENS.

14. If a medication is for ______________ use only, then the patient must be sure never to put the medication inside her body.

to affect	to achieve	potential	proper
strength	supine	evident	willingness
regarding	to maintain (maintenance)	absent	

1. If a patient is **unable** to stand, the therapist must do exercises with the patient in the _______________ position.

2. Pain is _______________ in patients with third degree **burns** because the nerve endings are destroyed.

3. When massaging an injured area, it is important to use the _______________ technique for the type of injury sustained.

4. One of the factors that influences the speed of a patient's recovery is his _______________ to work hard **during** physical therapy.

5. Resistance exercises are usually done with a patient **in order to increase** her muscle _______________.

6. The western medical world is now beginning to realize that a patient's attitude can greatly _______________ his chance and rate of recovery.

7. Exercise and a healthy diet are two important factors for _______________ your mental and physical health.

8. **After** testing the patient's gait, it was _______________ to the therapist that the patient would need extensive therapy.

9. To _______________ the best **results**, it is important for a patient to follow all of the instructions of the therapist.

10. An **innappropriate** question to ask your supervisor is one _______________ their salary.

11. _______________ is the ability to do or use something, but not actually doing or using it.

Chapter 11
Areas of Study

This list of important study areas will allow you to organize your studying time. We recommend that you study all of the sections, however we have placed stars (*) next to the areas that we believe are more important than others.

Note that each section also has a percentage next to the stars. This number represents the percentage of time we think you should spend for that particular area. Also, we have given separate stars and percentages for both PT and PTAs.

This outline is a way of directing your studies more efficiently. It is **not**, however, a complete guide of what you need to know. You must use your available physical therapy textbooks for the specific information suggested for study. You must also concentrate on the typical treatment procedures and goals for all areas.

OUTLINE CONTENTS

I. ANATOMY (PT)* **6%** (PTA)*** **15%**

A. Joints and Articulations

1. Lower Extremity
   - a. foot
   - b. ankle
   - c. knee
   - d. pelvic girdle

2. Upper Extremity
   - a. hand and fingers
   - b. wrist
   - c. elbow
   - d. shoulder girdle

B. Ligaments

1. ankle
2. knee
3. hip
4. elbow
5. shoulder

C. Muscle Actions

1. Lower Extremity
   - a. hip
   - b. knee
   - c. ankle

2. Upper Extremity
   - a. neck
   - b. scapula
   - c. shoulder
   - d. elbow and forearm
   - e. wrist
   - f. trunk and back

D. Vertebral Levels of Bony Landmarks

Levels	**Landmarks**
inferior angle of scapula	7th rib
iliac crest	L4, L5
sacroiliac joint	S2
spinal cord ends	L2
spine of scapula	T3
superior angle of scapula	2nd rib

E. Gross Anatomy

*You must know each muscle's *origin, insertion, innervation,* and *level* for the upper and lower extremities.

II. NEUROANATOMY (PT)* (6%) (PTA)*** (15%)

A. Cranial Nerves

nerve	type	function
I olfactory	sensory	smell
II optic	sensory	vision
III oculomotor	motor	eye movement
IV trochlear	motor	eyeball movement, pupil constriction
V trigeminal	motor, sensory	eyeball movement, facial sensations
VI abducens	motor	eye movement
VII facial	motor, sensory	facial movement, taste
VIII vestibulocochlear	sensory	hearing, balance
IX glossopharyngeal	motor, sensory	swallowing, taste
X vagus	motor, sensory	various movements, sensation from heart, larynx, trachea
XI accesory	motor	turning head, lifting shoulders
XII hypoglossal	motor	movement of tongue

B. Deep Tendon Reflexes

root level	muscle	peripheral nerve
C5-6	biceps	musculocutaneous
C5-6	brachioradialis	radial
C-7	triceps	radial
L3-4	quadriceps	femoral
S1	gastrocnemius	sciatic

III. MUSCLE TESTING (PT)*(6%) (PTA)*** (15%)

A. Grading System (Lovet Test)

B. Average Ranges of Motion

1. Upper Extremities
    a. shoulder
    b. elbow
    c. wrist

2. Lower Extremities
    a. hip
    b. knee
    c. ankle
    d. subtalar
    e. transverse tarsal
    f. toes
        1. first MTP
        2. first IP
        3. 2-5 MTP

4. PIP
5. DIP

g. cervical spine
h. thoracic and lumbar spine
i. temporomandibular

IV. MODALITIES (PT)* **6%** (PTA)* **5%**

*For each of the following modalities, you must know the *effects, indications, contraindications,* and *precautions.*

A. Heat
B. Ultrasound (0.8 to 3 MHz)
C. Phonophoresis
Phonophoresis is a process that delivers medicine into deep muscles and nerves by using ultrasound.
D. Cryotherapy (Ice Packs, Iced Towels, Ice Massage, Cold Baths [Immersion], Vapocoolant Spray, Contrast Baths)
E. Shortwave Diathermy
F. Hydrotherapy (Whirlpool and Hubbard Tank)
G. Ultraviolet Radiation
H. Intermittent Compression Pump
I. Direct Current- Ion Transfer
J. Mechanical Spinal Traction
K. Electrical Stimulation
L. Transcutaneous Electrical Nerve Stimulation (TENS)
M. High Voltage Pulsed Galvanic Stimulation (HVPGS)
N. Electromyographic Biofeedback
O. Inferential Stimulation

V. CHEST PHYSICAL THERAPY (ALL)*

A. Postural Drainage

A way of clearing the airways of secretions by placing the patient in certain positions so that gravity will help the flow of mucus

1. Indications
2. Contraindications
3. Contraindications
   a. upper lobes
   b. middle lobe
   c. lower lobes

B. Obstructive Pulmonary Diseases

1. Types
   a. chronic bronchitis
   b. emphysema
   c. asthma
   d. bronchiectasis
   e. cystic fibrosis

C. Restrictive Pulmonary Diseases

1. Types
   a. extrapulmonary restrictions
      1. pleural disease

2. chest wall injury or stiffness (scoliosis, scleroderma, etc.)
3. respiratory muscle weakness (neuromuscular disease, CNS injury)
4. obesity or ascites

b. pulmonary restrictions

1. tumor
2. atelectasis
3. pneumonia
4. heart disease

VI. PROSTHETICS (PT)** 10% (PTA) 5%

A. Levels of Amputation in the Lower Extremities
B. Common Reasons for Amputations
C. Postoperative Complications and Problems
D. Contractures
1. Above Knee Amputations
2. Below Knee Amputations
E. Gait Deviations (And Possible Causes)
1. Below-Knee Prosthetic
2. Above-Knee Prosthetic

VII. ORTHOTICS (PT)** 10% (PTA)* 5%

A. Definition

An orthosis is an external appliance used to restrict or enhance a body motion or function. An orthosis is also used to reduce the load on a particular body part.

B. Types of Orthosis
1. Ankle-foot
2. Knee-ankle
3. Lumbosacral
4. Thoracolumbar
5. Cervical

VIII. ORTHOPEDICS (PT)** 10% (PTA) 5%

A. Tests Used for Injury Diagnosis

1. *Adson test*-determines the presence of thoracic outlet syndrome
2. *Anterior/posterior draw test*- tests the stability of the anterior and posterior knee ligament
3. *Apply compression test*- helps to diagnose a torn meniscus
4. *Apprehension test for shoulder dislocation*- test for chronic shoulder dislocation
5. *Drop arm test*-tests if there is a tear in the supraspinatus muscle
6. *Lachman test*-tests the stability of the anterior cruciate ligament
7. *Mcmurray test*-tests the stability of the menisci
8. *Ober test*-tests for a tight or contracted iliotibial band
9. *Patella femoral grinding test*- tests the status of the patella where it articulates with the trochlear groove of the femur
10. *Phalen's test*-tests for carpal tunnel syndrome
11. *Thomas' test*-tests for a flexion contracture of the hip
12. *Thompson test*-tests if the achilles tendon is ruptured
13. *Tinel's sign*-test to elicit tenderness over a neuroma within a nerve
14. *Varus/valgus test*-tests the stability of the knee ligaments
15. *Yergason's test*-tests whether the bicep tendon is stable within the bicipital groove

IX. PEDIATRICS (PT)** 10% (PTA)* 5%

A. Growth and Development (through age 4)
   *You must know the characteristics of normal child development for each month of the first 1.5 years and then for each year after.

B. Developmental Reflexes
   *For each of the developmental reflexes, you must know the *stimulus* and *response*
   1. Spinal Reflexes
   2. Brainstem Reflexes
   3. Midbrain/Cortical Reflexes

X. GAIT (PT)** 10% (PTA)* 5%

A. Definitions
   1. Stance Phase
   2. Swing Phase

B. Normal Values
   1. Cadence-120 steps per minute
   2. Step Length-15 inches
   3. Base of Support-1-5 inches
   4. Degree of Toe Out-7 degrees

C. Gait Deviations

XI. CARDIOLOGY (PT)** 10% (PTA)* 5%

A. Anatomy of the Heart

B. Blood Pressure
   1. Normal blood pressure
   2. Hypertension

C. Heart Rate
   1. Normal Heart Rate
   2. Maximal Heart Rate
   3. Bradycardia
   4. Tachycardia

D. Stages for Patients with Cardiopulmonary History and/or Precautions
   1. Stage I (1.0-1.4 METs) (METs=Metabolic Equivalents)
   2. Stage II (1.4- 2.0 METs)
   3. Stage III (2.0- 3.0 METs)
   4. Stage IV (3.0- 3.5 METs)
   5. Stage V (3.5- 4.0 METs)
   6. Stage VI (4.0- 5.0 METs)

XII. CLINICAL DISORDERS (PT)** 10% (PTA)*** 15%

*For each of the following disorders, you must know the *characteristics* and *treatment*.

A. Bell's Palsy
B. Buerger's Disease (Thromboangitis Obliterans)
C. Chondromalacia
D. Cushing's Disease
E. Cystic Fibrosis
F. Diabetes Mellitus
G. Down's Syndrome
H. Emphysema

I. Guillain-Barre Syndrome
J. Hodgkin's Disease
K. Huntington's Chorea
L. Marfan's Syndrome
M. Multiple Sclerosis
N. Muscular Dystrophy
O. Myasthenia Gravis
P. Osgood-Schlatter Disease
Q. Osteoporosis
R. Parkinson's Disease
S. Scleroderma
T. Thrombus

Chapter 12
PT Practice Exam

1. While observing a patient with a left below knee amputation you notice that during the late stance phase of gait the patient shows delayed knee flexion. All of the following are possible causes of this condition except:
A. socket positioned too far posteriorly
B. socket positioned too far anteriorly
C. extensor spasticity
D. excessive plantarflexion

2. Physical therapy departments keep departmental records for all of the following reasons except:
A. organizational efficiency
B. to maintain high standards of therapy care
C. department planning
D. to avoid malpractice lawsuits

3. A 55-year-old office administrator was referred for home health physical therapy after suffering a myocardial infarction. The patient is very eager to improve quickly and wants to return to normal daily activities as soon as possible. During treatment, it is important to:
A. monitor vital signs
B. educate the patient and family regarding treatment
C. modify treatment as patient progresses
D. all of the above

4. A patient needs to increase his range of motion of a muscle. You can use hold-relax or contract-relax technique. What is the main difference between these two techniques?
A. isotonic contractions
B. passive patient participation
C. direction of movement
D. none of the above

5. A 25-year-old male who was involved in a car accident has sustained a C6 spinal cord injury. As the patient's therapist, you have already done an initial evaluation and are now writing the long-term goals. All of the following long-term goals are appropriate for this type of injury except:
A. independent transfer with sliding board
B. independent bed mobility
C. independent skin inspection
D. independent shoe tying

6. A 65-year-old retired piano teacher is referred to you for physical therapy. The following symptoms are observed in the patient: morning stiffness, weakness of the hands, mallet finger deformity, and skin irritation around the joint areas. From these symptoms, you should expect that the patient is suffering from:
A. rheumatoid arthritis
B. bursitis
C. multiple sclerosis
D. carpal tunnel syndrome

7. You are assigned by the director of your physical therapy department to redesign the physical therapy department. Which of the following is the least important factor to consider?
A. current number of staff physical therapists
B. the size of the hospital
C. changes in practice
D. source of referrals

8. You are training a patient to use a pick-up walker with partial weight bearing on the right lower extremity. Which gait sequence would you use?
A. walker pushed forward, right lower extremity moved forward, left lower extremity moved forward
B. walker picked up and moved forward, right lower extremity moved forward, left lower extremity moved forward
C. walker picked up and moved forward, left lower extremity moved forward, right lower extremity moved forward
D. right lower extremity moved forward, walker picked up and moved forward, left lower extremity moved forward

9. When doing a quality assurance program, it is important to do an outcome assessment based on the condition of the patient during which of the following times?
A. at the time of evaluation
B. during the patient's treatment period
C. at the end of care period
D. after discharge

10. You are treating a patient with a Syme's amputation. As a therapist, you should know that the level of the patient's amputation is:
A. the foot at the supramalleolar level
B. the foot at the midtarsal joint
C. the femur from the pelvis
D. none of the above

11. As a physical therapist working in the acute care department, you are treating a patient with a cerebral artery occlusion. The patient shows hemiplegia in the lower extremity, aphasia, confusion, and hemianesthesia. From these symptoms, you should conclude that the involved artery is:
A. middle cerebral
B. anterior cerebral
C. posterior cerebral
D. vertebral-basilar

12. Which of the following spinal reflexes normally continue on throughout the entire growth process?
A. moro
B. grasp
C. startle
D. traction

13. All of the following are typical, realistic goals for a C-8 spinal cord victim except:
A. ambulation with bilateral knee-ankle orthosis and crutches
B. driving with hand controls
C. able to work
D. independent in all self-care

14. Which of the following differences are found between the cerebral stretch reflex and the spinal cord stretch reflex?
A. the gamma-efferent fibers are used only in the spinal cord stretch reflex
B. in the cerebeller stretch reflex, impulses arising from the muscle spindles pass through the brain stem to the cerebral fastigial nuclei
C. the feedback time of the cerebral stretch reflex is much longer
D. all of the above are differences

15. You have received a physician's order to perform mobilization techniques for a patient with a right shoulder sprain. What position should the shoulder be placed in while performing the inferior glide of the humeral head?
A. abducted to 30 degrees
B. slight flexion
C. externally rotated
D. internally rotated

16. When treating a person with multiple sclerosis, there are certain factors that determine whether the prognosis for the patient will be favorable. All of the following are factors which determine the prognosis except:
A. age of onset
B. neurologic status at 5 years
C. rate of onset
D. all of the above

17. A 65-year-old male has suffered a stroke, and has been referred to you for physical therapy. The patient is able to walk, shows good balance, and understands your directions, however he is unable to produce normal speech sounds. Which of the following terms is used to describe this patient's problem?
A. agnosia
B. apraxia
C. aphonia
D. asthenia

18. Which of the following are indications for using electromyography?
A. chronaxie
B. fibrillation voltage
C. rheobase
D. none of the above

19. A 32-year-old woman diagnosed with cancer has had an above right knee amputation. During gait training, the patient begins to complain of stump pain. Your immediate response should be to:
A. tell the patient that the pain is normal and she should continue treatment
B. let the patient rest and continue the treatment after a short while
C. remove the prosthesis and check the stump
D. call your supervisor

20. A patient has been diagnosed with pulmonary edema. After your initial evaluation, you find that the patient does not show signs of edema in the lower extremities. This would best indicate that the patient is suffering from which type of heart disease?
A. left ventricular
B. left atrium
C. right atrium
D. right ventricular

21. While working as a pediatric physical therapist, you are treating a 3-year-old child who is afflicted with cystic fibrosis. You should know that the primary area affected by this disease is the:
A. spleen
B. kidneys
C. heart
D. pancreas

22. A 55-year-old patient has been referred to physical therapy with a diagnosis of bronchiectasis. During the course of treatment, the patient and his family seem unclear about the details of this disease. You tell them that:
A. this is a restrictive lung disorder
B. this is a chronic bronchitis problem
C. this disease is a chronic dilation of the bronchi and bronchioles
D. this disease affects the upper lobes of the lungs most often

23. All of the following complications are results of a fracture except:
A. crush syndrome
B. contracture
C. loss of muscle strength
D. fat embolism

24. A 25-year-old woman involved in a car accident has been diagnosed with a fracture of the right clavicle. The patient complains of pain, swelling, numbness, and weakness in the right upper extremity. As her physical therapist, you should suspect that one of the possible causes for these symptoms could be:
A. Von Recklinghausen's Syndrome
B. thoracic outlet syndrome
C. carpal tunnel syndrome
D. Volkmann's Syndrome

25. All of the following are symptoms of AIDS except:
A. general weakness
B. skin irritation
C. pulmonary complications
D. all of the above

26. While working in an acute care unit as a physical therapist, you receive an order to treat a 25-year-old male who has been involved in an automobile accident. He has been diagnosed with a closed head injury. On the referral, it is listed that the patient has been diagnosed as HIV+. You do not wish to treat this patient because of the possibility of contracting AIDS. You tell your supervisor how you feel, but the supervisor tells you that you should continue treatment. What would be an appropriate response?
A. treat the patient
B. treat the patient, but report the incident to the physical therapy director
C. ask one of your co-workers to treat the patient
D. refuse to treat the patient, but report the incident to the physical therapy director

27. You are treating a 20-year-old man who sustained a shoulder injury while playing baseball. On his physical therapy referral you see that the patient has a tear in the supraspinatus muscle. What is the most appropriate test to use on this patient?
A. drop-arm test
B. Yergason Test
C. Tinel Sign
D. Phalen's Test

28. You are treating a 45-year-old male who has sustained a cerebral vascular accident. You want to improve trunk control, as the patient shows poor control of trunk mobility. Which of the following PNF techniques would you use?
A. traction
B. rhythmic stabilization
C. tonic holding
D. cocontraction

29. Spina bifida is one of the more common congential disorders. Clinical findings of this birth defect might include all of the following except:
A. normal lamina and spinous processes of one or more vertebrae
B. incomplete closure of the neural plate
C. severe paralysis
D. excretory dysfunctions

30. You are treating a 32-year-old male with a left above knee amputation who is full weight bearing, and you are giving instructions on the proper stair climbing method for ascending while using axillary crutches. Which of the following climbing sequences is correct for this patient?
A. right lower extremity up, left lower extremity up, right crutch up, left crutch up
B. left lower extremity up, right lower extremity up, left crutch up, right crutch up
C. right lower extremity up, left lower extremity up, left crutch up, right crutch up
D. left lower extremity up, right lower extremity up, right crutch up, left crutch up

31. A 55-year-old male with diabetes is referred to you for therapy following an above knee left lower extremity amputation as a result of poor circulation. As the patient's therapist, you are assessing the patient and determining the long term goals. Which of the following are valid long term goals for this patient?
A. independent in all ambulation and self-care activities
B. independent in bed mobility and transfer
C. prevent the development of joint contractures
D. maintain or regain strength in the affected lower extremity

32. A physical therapist must deal with many different types of medical records. One of these is the problem-oriented medical record. This type of record is used for all of the following purposes except:
A. organizing data
B. preserving medical logic
C. assessing quality care
D. restrict structure of care

33. A 65-year-old female with a history of diabetes, cardiovascular disease, and peripheral vascular disease has been referred to you for physical therapy after a right below knee amputation due to gangrene. She was fitted for a temporary prosthesis after the wound healed. There are many advantages to using a temporary prosthesis. All of the following are advantages to using a temporary prosthesis except:
A. shrinks the residual limb more effectively than elastic wrap
B. allows early bipedal ambulation
C. provide a better quality prosthesis
D. all of the above

34. You are treating a 32-year-old male with a closed head injury suffered while playing ice hockey. The patient is responding to treatment very well, however, you still want to improve his controlled mobility. Some therapeutic techniques that can enhance controlled mobility include all of the following except:
A. slow reversals
B. repeated contractions
C. resisted progression
D. slow reversal-hold

35. You are designing a cardiac program for a patient who has unstable angina and you are considering the patient's safe workload. Under which of the following situations can heart rate be used to prescribe this safe workload?
A. isotometric exercise
B. isotonic exercise
C. Valsalva maneuver
D. heavy arm work

36. You are treating a 45-year-old patient with a chronic heart disease. Before doing exercises, it is important to do warm-up activities. These activities promote the adjustments that the body must make before doing strenuous activity. Specifically, the warm-up period:
A. decreases venous return
B. decreases need for oxygen
C. increases muscle temperature
D. increases heart rate to within 40 beats per minute of target heart rate

37. When treating a patient who has recently undergone an amputation, what things must you be sure to check for to be certain that the prosthesis has been properly fitted?
A. discoloration
B. proper weight bearing
C. height of the posterior wall of the socket
D. all of the above

38. What is the average resting heart rate for infants?
A. 126 for girls, 135 for boys
B. 220 minus infant's age
C. 180 for girls, 190 for boys
D. the average resting heart rate for infants is the same as for adults

39. A 25-year-old female suffered a subluxation of the radial head as a result of a fall taken while walking her dog. Given what you know about this condition, commonly known as "pushed elbow", what clinical findings would you expect to see in this patient?
A. the radial head is pushed distally in the annular ligament
B. occurs as a result of a fall on the shoulder
C. occurs as a result of a fall on the outstretched hand
D. all of the above are common clinical findings

40. Postoperative edema is one of the complications that may occur following an amputation. One of the ways of treating this problem is by the use of rigid dressing. Althought this method is effective, it does have certain disadvantages compared to more traditional soft dressing. All of the following are disadvantages of rigid dressing except:
A. requires close supervision during healing stage
B. daily wound inspection not possible
C. causes delayed ambulation
D. requires technical skills to apply

41. A 72-year-old male patient is referred to you for physical therapy treatment after having a fall and fracturing his hip. The patient had an open reduction and internal fixation of the hip. In order to achieve normal hip functioning, all of the following goals must be accomplished except:
A. no pain in the hip
B. stable extremity for weight bearing
C. full range of motion and strength
D. use of an assistive device

42. You are modifying the cardiac program of a 44-year-old male who is receiving therapy as a result of a left ventricular dysfunction. All of the following factors must be carefully considered when making this change except:
A. patient's age
B. health status
C. motivation
D. patient's insurance coverage

43. All of the following are typical causes of chondromalacia patellae except:
A. prolonged or repeated stress
B. surgery
C. trauma
D. virus

44. All of the following are components of a knee prosthesis except:
A. axis
B. fork strap
C. friction brake
D. all of the above are components of the knee prosthesis

45. A 16-year-old patient sustained an acute sprain and partial tear of the ligaments in his knee while playing volleyball. Which of the following methods of treatment would be most appropriate for this patient?
A. rest
B. joint protection
C. gentle exercises
D. all of the above are appropriate

46. You are treating a 38-year-old woman suffering from multiple sclerosis. After initial evaluation, you find many abnormalities. Which of the following symptoms should you expect to find in a person diagnosed with multiple sclerosis?
A. motor weakness
B. diplopia
C. ataxic gait
D. all of the above

47. While treating a patient with a denervated muscle, it is important to consider all of the following factors except:
A. frequency
B. patient's age
C. duration
D. intensity

48. As a therapist working in an outpatient clinic, you are treating a patient with tendinitis of the long head of the biceps brachii muscle. If you want to gain a full internal rotation and flexion of the shoulder, which glide would be most appropriate for this patient?
A. posterior glide
B. anterior glide
C. anterior glide progression
D. caudal glide

49. A 17-year-old male has suffered a head injury as a result of a motorcycle accident. During the acute stage of recovery, you decide to use the Glasgow Coma Scale. This scale rates which of the following responses?
A. eye opening, sensation response, pain response
B. eye opening, best motor response, verbal response
C. eye opening, sensation response, verbal response
D. eye opening, reflex response, verbal response

50. A 25-year-old female patient has suffered a severe head injury during a car accident. During your initial evaluation, the family begins to question you on the rate and amount of recovery they can expect from the patient. You should tell the family that the majority of recovery will take place:
A. within the first month
B. within the first 3 months
C. within the first 6 months
D. within the first year

51. Which of the following is the correct definition for a second-degree burn?
A. damage through the dermal layer
B. damage to the epidermal layer
C. damage to the epidermal and part of dermal layer
D. none of the above are correct definitions of second-degree burns

52. You are treating a 32-year-old patient who has recently sprained his ankle. You decide that cryotherapy is the form of treatment you wish to use. Which of the following is an effect of cryotherapy?
A. increase in local metabolism
B. increase in local perspiration
C. promotion of muscle relaxation
D. decrease in local metabolism

53. You are treating a patient with a peripheral vascular disease. You are ordered by the physician to use diathermy. You should be aware that the most appropriate length of treatment using diathermy for this condition is:
A. 5 minutes
B. 5 to 10 minutes
C. 20 to 30 minutes
D. 30 to 40 minutes

54. Which of the following are different names for the simple stretch reflex?
A. patellar tendon reflex
B. myostatic reflex
C. flexor withdrawal reflex
D. both A and B

55. What is unique or different about the cortical control of muscle function?
A. this control is learned
B. this control is voluntary
C. this control is autonomic
D. this control is integrated

56. A patient who has sustained a right knee sprain is referred to you for physical therapy. After several weeks of treatment, the patient still complains of pain. You decide to use ultrasound to treat this patient. What wattage would you use to increase the nerve conduction velocity?
A. 1 Watt/ cm2
B. 1.5 Watt/ cm2
C. 3 Watt/ cm2
D. both A and B are acceptable wattages

57. As a physical therapist, you know that you can increase pulmonary diffusion capacity during exercises. All of the following are causes of this except:
A. increase in tidal volume
B. a greater pulmonary vasodilation
C. a decrease in the functional residual volume
D. a pulmonary capillary blood volume which is double that of the resting state

58. Scoliosis is a spinal defect which causes postural deformity. In order to measure the amount of spinal curvature, there are many types of tests available. Which of the following is a type of measurement test of spinal curvature?
A. Master's test
B. Kerring test
C. C'obb method
D. Hoover method

59. You are treating a 75-year-old female who sustained a right hip fracture. She is currently full weight bearing and her upper extremity strength is grossly fair plus. Which assistive device would be most appropriate for this patient?
A. large base support quad cane
B. small base support quad cane
C. crutches
D. wheeled walker

60. When you are working with geriatric patients, it is important to keep in mind that certain exercises don't need to be focused on. All of the following exercises should be focused on with geriatric patients except:
A. hip flexion
B. hip extension
C. knee extension
D. knee flexion

61. There are many deformities related to rheumatoid arthritis. One of these deformities is known as a boutonniere deformity. The characteristics of this affliction are:
A. DIP hyperextension with PIP flexion
B. DIP flexion with PIP hyperextension
C. DIP flexion with PIP extension
D. DIP extension with PIP flexion

62. A 55-year-old female has been referred for physical therapy. She shows the following symptoms: mutilans type deformity, hammer toes, exostoses, and pannus. Based on this information, this patient is probably suffering from:
A. Parkinson's disease
B. rheumatoid arthritis
C. multiple sclerosis
D. arthritis

63. Parkinson's disease is a progressive disease which affects males more often than females. What are the major central nervous system structures involved in this disease?
A. spinal cord
B. pons
C. thalamus
D. none of the above

64. A 16-year-old female has suffered a second degree burn on her hip and groin and has been referred for treatment. Which of the following positions would be appropriate for this patient to avoid contracture?
A. hip neutral with slight abduction
B. hip slightly flexed (10 degrees)
C. hip slightly flexed (5 degrees) and slight adduction
D. hip neutral with slight adduction

65. Rehabilitation goals for a 52-year-old high school basketball coach diagnosed with chronic heart disease include all of the following except:
A. good breathing and coughing
B. prevention of venous stasis
C. return to competitive athletics
D. control of anxiety and tension

66. You are treating a spinal cord injury victim who has an autonomous or nonreflexive bladder. To empty this patient's bladder, you must increase intra-abdominal pressure using which kind of technique?
A. Brown-Sequard maneuver
B. Valsalva maneuver
C. Williams maneuver
D. airshift maneuver

67. A 6-month-old infant is referred to you for therapy to treat his condition of hydrocephalus. This condition is most often caused by:
A. obstruction of the flow of cerebral spinal fluid
B. congenital ventricular hypertrophy
C. obstruction of blood circulation to the brain
D. both B and C

68. A 25-year-old male jumped off of a bridge into shallow water causing a T-9 spinal cord injury. The patient has shown an intense motivation to be able to walk again, and asks you if you believe he will be able to do so. The most appropriate response to this patient's question is:
A. yes, but only a short distance with a walker
B. yes, but only a short distance with crutches
C. yes, but only a short distance with crutches and knee-ankle-foot orthosis
D. yes, but only a short distance with crutches and ankle-foot orthosis

69. Which of the following definitions best describe a complete lesion in a spinal cord injury?
A. some sensory or motor function below the level of the lesion
B. no motor function below the level of the lesion
C. no sensory or motor function below the level of the lesion
D. none of the above

70. While teaching patients breathing excercises for their home programs, what should you tell the patients to avoid doing?
A. do not force expiration
B. do not take a prolonged expiration
C. do not initiate inspiration with the upper chest
D. all of the above

71. Asthma is an obstructive lung disease most often seen in a young patient. All of the following are accurate clinical pictures of this affliction except:
A. rounded shoulders
B. abnormal breathing pattern
C. chronic fatigue
D. exocrine gland dysfunction

72. You are treating a 30-year-old female patient who has chronic lower back pain. The attending physician has ordered ultrasound treatment, however because the patient is 4 months pregnant, you know that ultrasound should not be used. The appropriate response in this situation is to:
A. continue treatment as ordered
B. use hot packs instead of ultrasound
C. tell the patient that the doctor made a mistake and you cannot use ultrasound
D. call the doctor and discuss the situation

73. When testing the range of motion for the hip, there are possible capsular patterns of restrictive motion. Which of the following capsular patterns are typical for the hip?
A. minimal loss of internal rotation, maximal loss of flexion and abduction
B. minimal loss of internal rotation, maximal loss of exension and adduction
C. maximal loss of internal rotation, flexion, abduction, minimal loss of extension
D. maximal loss of external rotation, extension, adduction, minimal loss of flexion

74. An 18-year-old patient with a fractured left femur is non-weight bearing and needs physical therapy. You decide to use axillary crutches for gait training. What is the appropriate method for measuring these crutches?
A. while standing, the crutches should be 2 inches below the axilla and the distal end of the crutch should be 2 inches lateral and 6 inches anterior to the foot
B. while standing, the crutches should be 6 inches below the axilla and the distal end of the crutch should be 4 inches lateral and 4 inches anterior to the foot
C. while standing, the crutches should be directly under the axilla and the distal end of the crutch should be 3 inches lateral and 2 inches anterior to the foot
D. while standing, the crutches should be 4 inches below the axilla and the distal end of the crutch should be 4 inches lateral and 4 inches anterior to the foot.

75. One of the complications of a spinal cord injury is autonomic hyperreflexia.This condition could not occur in a patient with which level of spinal cord injury?
A. C-3
B. T-1
C. T-4
D. L-2

76. You are treating a 65-year-old stroke patient. This patient demonstrates severe synergy patterns of the right upper extremity. The typical extension synergy components for the shoulder is:
A. scapular retraction, shoulder abduction, elbow flexion, wrist and finger flexion
B. scapular protraction, shoulder abduction, elbow extension, forearm pronation, finger flexion
C. scapular protraction, shoulder adduction, internal rotation, elbow extension, forearm pronation, finger flexion
D. scapular protraction, shoulder adduction, external rotation, elbow flexion, forearm pronation, finger flexion

77. You are designing a study to measure the effect of heat used to remove a patient's pain. In this study, what is heat considered?
A. dependent variable
B. independent variable
C. hypothesis
D. control group

78. A 10-year-old child is being treated for lumbar lordosis. Which of the following spinal orthoses would you use to treat this problem?
A. Tyler's brace
B. Oswald's brace
C. Milwaukee brace
D. William's brace

79. You are working as a staff physical therapist in a large hospital. While on lunch break break one day, you read a notice that says there is an opening for the physical therapist supervisor position. To be an effective leader of a physical therapy department, it is important to have all of the following skills except:
A. ability to resolve conflicts well
B. ability to encourage the creativity of the staff
C. ability to work overtime hours
D. ability to develop the staff's abilities

80. As a therapist assigned to treating a patient with uremic pruritis, you are ordered to use ultraviolet radiation for treatment. All of the following are contraindications for ultraviolet radiation except:
A. pressure sores
B. fever
C. cardiac disease
D. patients involved in x-ray therapy

81. During the swing phase of normal gait, you should expect that the biceps femoris muscle:
A. has no activity
B. contracts concentrically
C. contracts eccentrically
D. both B and C

82. Which of the following conditions is not important when observing gait?
A. area in which the patient will walk
B. previous selection of joint or segment to be observed
C. select a plane observation
D. patient's weight

83. A typical complication for a head injury patient is spasticity. One of the most effective forms of treatment for this problem is:
A. resistive exercises
B. casting
C. phenol blocks
D. electrostimulation

84. Which of the following possible causes are indicative of the toe clawing gait deviation during stance phase?
A. spastic toe flexors
B. flaccidity of plantarflexion
C. diminished hip flexion
D. diminished hamstring action

85. All of the following proprioceptive stimulation techniques inhibit muscle response except:
A. quick stretch
B. prolonged stretch
C. high frequency vibration
D. prolonged icing

86. While treating patients with total hip replacements, during the first few weeks following the operation it is important to avoid all of the following actions except:
A. isometric exercises
B. hip flexion beyond 90 degrees
C. hip adduction across the midline
D. avoid excessive bending of the trunk over the hip

87. Which of the following behaviors would you expect to see in a normal 3 month old child?
A. head held steady while moving
B. reaches for object with one hand
C. sits without support
D. sits down

88. Sensations transmitted by the dorsal column-medial lemniscal pathway include all of the following except:
A. stereognosis
B. hyperalgesia
C. barognosis
D. two-point discrimination

89. When designing a wheelchair for a patient, it is important to correctly measure the patient to insure a proper fit. To determine the proper height of the foot plate, for example, the patient is measured:
A. from the popliteal fossa to the bottom of the heel
B. from the iliac crest to the bottom of the heel
C. from the trochanter major to the bottom of the heel
D. from the midback to the bottom of the heel

90. While teaching a patient with a knee-ankle foot orthosis to climb the stairs, you observe knee instability. All of the following are possible causes of this gait deviation except:
A. inadequate knee lock
B. knee flexion contracture
C. weak abductors
D. weak quadriceps

91. You are doing the daily documentation for your home health care patient who is recovering from stroke. The patient comments to you that he is having a good day and seems happy. Which section of the "SOAP" note would you place this entry?
A. objective
B. subjective
C. assessment
D. plan

92. After an amputation, there are many complications and problems that a patient must overcome. One of the most common psychological problems is that the patient continues to feel the removed extremity even though it is no longer there. This condition is known as:
A. myodesis
B. phantom limb
C. stubbies
D. none of the above

93. Physical therapist assistants can do all of the following except:
A. administer therapeutic modalities
B. measure muscle strength
C. modify treatment plan
D. measure range of motion

94. Mechanical spinal traction is used to reduce signs or symptoms of cervical lumbar spinal compression. Which of the following are contraindications for mechanical spinal traction:
A. meningitis
B. herniation
C. protrusion
D. spinal stenosis

95. A patient who is 3 days status post total knee replacement is receiving treatment from you. The physician has ordered the use of continuous passive motion as a treatment method. One of the advantages of this type of treatment is:
A. decrease contracture formation
B. decrease postoperative pain
C. decrease joint effusion
D. all of the above

96. All of the following are characteristics of agnosia except:
A. simultagnosia
B. prosopagnosia
C. ideognosia
D. color agnosia

97. You are a home health care therapist visiting your patient at the scheduled time and date. When you arrive at the patient's home, you find that a nurse's aide has just begun to prepare the patient for a bath. What is the most appropriate response?
A. tell the nurse's aide to stop her activities and wait until you have finished your treatment
B. tell the patient that you can't wait for him and you will reschedule for another day
C. call your supervisor and explain the problem
D. tell the patient that they will have to miss this visit and you will be back for the next regularly scheduled visit

98. Carpal tunnel syndrome involves intrinsic muscles of the thenar eminence and lumbricals. Which of the following nerves are involved with this condition?
A. ulnar nerve
B. median nerve
C. thoracic nerve
D. radial nerve

99. Multiple sclerosis is a demyelinating disease of the central nervous system that is not yet curable. This disease is most often seen in:
A. young adult females
B. young adult males
C. children
D. none of the above

100. While you are treating a patient who has sustained a head injury while playing football, you observe that the patient has a tendency to cross the midline during his gait. As a physical therapist assistant, you can classify this gait pattern as:
A. spastic
B. scissor
C. gluteal
D. tabetic

Chapter 13
PTA Practice Exam

1. The most appropriate position to test the strength of the patient's sternocleidomastoid muscle is:
A. patient standing
B. patient sitting
C. patient supine
D. patient prone

2. Physical therapy departments keep records for all of the following reasons except:
A. organizational efficiency
B. to maintain high standards of therapy care
C. department planning
D. to avoid malpractice law suits

3. A physical therapist assistant performs a manual muscle test on the gastrocnemius and soleus muscles. What is the appropriate postition for the patient with a fair grade muscle strength?
A. sidelying
B. sitting
C. prone
D. standing on limb to be tested

4. You are a physical therapist assistant treating a 32-year-old male patient with tension of the dorsiflexor muscle of the ankle. You perform goniometric measurements to test the patient's range of motion and the results were 0 to 25 degrees plantarflexion. Based on this information, what can you conclude about the patient's ankle?
A. the ankle has limited range of motion
B. the ankle has functional range of motion
C. there is not enough information to determine anything
D. none of the above

5. A 55-year-old office administrator was referred for home health physical therapy after suffering a myocardial infarction. The patient is very eager to improve quickly and wants to return to normal daily activities as soon as possible. During treatment, it is important to:
A. monitor vital signs
B. educate the patient and family regarding treatment
C. modify treatment as patient progresses
D. all of the above

6. All of the following muscles are active during ankle eversion except:
A. peroneus longus
B. peroneus brevis
C. tibialis posterior
D. peroneus tertius

7. A 25-year-old male who was involved in a car accident has sustained a C6 spinal cord injury. The patient's therapist has already done an initial evaluation and is now writing the long-term goals. All of the following long-term goals are appropriate for this type of injury except:
A. independent transfer with sliding board
B. independent bed mobility
C. independent skin inspection
D. independent shoe tying

8. You are a physical therapist assistant working in an outpatient clinic and your supervisor asks you to test the rectus abdominus muscle strength of a patient who is suffering from chronic lower back pain. What is the most appropriate position to test this muscle for the normal grade of strength?
A. supine, with patient's hands behind his neck
B. prone, with patient's hands behind his neck
C. standing, with patient's arms at his sides
D. sitting, with patient's hands behind his neck

9. A patient needs to increase her range of motion of a muscle. You can use hold-relax or contract-relax technique. What is the main difference between these two techniques?
A. isotonic contractions
B. verbal comments
C. direction of movement
D. none of the above

10. A 35-year-old female has been referred for physical therapy after a left femur fracture. The patient complains of hip pain, and after speaking with your supervisor, you are instructed to take a goniometric measurement of the medial rotation of the hip. Which of the following locations would be most appropriate for the placement of the goniometer while testing the patient in the sitting position?
A. directly below the patella
B. anterior aspect of the patella
C. midline of the lower leg
D. directly above the patella

11. A 65-year-old retired piano teacher is referred to you for physical therapy. The following symptoms are observed in the patient: morning stiffness, weakness of the hands, mallet finger deformity, and skin irritation around the joint areas. From these symptoms, you should expect that the patient is suffering from:
A. rheumatoid arthritis
B. bursitis
C. multiple sclerosis
D. carpal tunnel syndrome

12. Which of the following spinal reflexes normally continue on throughout the entire growth process?
A. moro
B. grasp
C. startle
D. traction

13. As a physical therapist assistant, you should know that during a goniometric measurement the following sequence should be followed:
A. stabilize proximal joint component, place a joint at zero degrees, permit complete range of motion
B. place a joint at zero degrees, permit complete range of motion, stabilize proximal joint component
C. stabilize proximal joint component, permit complete range of motion, place a joint at zero degrees
D. place a joint at zero degrees, stabilize proximal joint component, permit complete range of motion

14. You are training a patient to use a pick-up walker with partial weight bearing on the right lower extremity. Which gait sequence would you use?
A. walker pushed forward, right lower extremity moved forward, left lower extremity moved forward
B. walker picked up and moved forward, right lower extremity moved forward, left lower extremity moved forward
C. walker picked up and moved forward, left lower extremity moved forward, right lower extremity moved forward
D. right lower extremity moved forward, walker picked up and moved forward, left lower extremity moved forward

15. What is a normal range of motion for the eversion of the foot?
A. 0 to 5 degrees
B. 5 to 10 degrees
C. 0 to 15 degrees
D. 0 to 20 degrees

16. You are treating a patient with a Syme's amputation. As a therapist, you should know that the level of the patient's amputation is:
A. the foot at the supramalleolar level
B. the foot at the midtarsal joint
C. the femur from the pelvis
D. none of the above

17. You are testing the muscle strength of the flexor digitorium brevis of a patient who sustained an ankle sprain. What is the correct origin of this muscle?
A. medial process of tuberosity of calcaneus
B. posterior process of tuberosity of calcaneus
C. anterior process of tuberosity of calcaneus
D. lateral process of tuberosity of calcaneus

18. You are treating a patient who has sustained a knee injury while playing tennis. You would like to improve the patient's muscle strength of the knee flexors. The semitendinosus is one of these knee flexors. As a physical therapist assistant, you should know that the insertion of this muscle is at the:
A. distal part of the anteromedial surface of the tibia
B. proximal part of the anteromedial surface of the tibia
C. proximal part of the posteriomedial surface of the tibia
D. distal part of the posteriomedial surface of the tibia

19. All of the following are typical realistic goals for a C-8 spinal cord patient except:
A. ambulation with bilateral knee-ankle orthosis and crutches
B. driving with hand controls
C. able to work
D. independent in all self-care

20. You are treating a patient with a second degree hip sprain injury. During treatment, the patient has difficulty performing lateral rotation of the hip. You could suspect that all of the following muscles might be weak except:
A. quadriceps femoris
B. piriformis
C. gluteus medius
D. obturator externus

21. When treating a person with multiple sclerosis, there are certain factors that determine whether the prognosis for the patient will be favorable. All of the following are factors which determine the prognosis except:
A. age of onset
B. neurologic status at 5 years
C. rate of onset
D. all of the above

22. While you are taking a goniometric measurement of knee flexion, where do you place the stationary arm of the goniometer?
A. posterior longitudinal midline of the thigh
B. anterior longitudinal midline of the thigh
C. in front of the patella
D. lateral longitudinal midline of the thigh

23. A physical therapist has made an initial evaluation for a patient who sustained a fracture of the talus. The therapist has requested that you test the muscle strength of the ankle plantarflexors. All of the following muscles provide plantarflexion for the ankle except:
A. gastrocnemius
B. tibialis anterior
C. soleus
D. peroneus longus

24. You wish to take the measurement of lateral flexion of the trunk. As a physical therapist assistant, you know that you should stabilize the pelvis in order to:
A. prevent anterior tilting
B. prevent posterior tilting
C. prevent lateral tilting
D. prevent hip action

25. A 65-year-old male has suffered a stroke, and has been referred to you for physical therapy. The patient is able to walk, shows good balance, and understands your directions, however he is unable to produce normal speech sounds. Which of the following terms is used to describe this patient's problem?
A. agnosia
B. apraxia
C. aphonia
D. asthenia

26. A 32-year-old woman diagnosed with cancer has had an above right knee amputation. During gait training, the patient begins to complain of stump pain. Your immediate response should be to:
A. tell the patient that the pain is normal and she should continue treatment
B. let the patient rest and continue the treatment after a short while
C. remove the prosthesis and check the stump
D. call your supervisor

27. While working as a pediatric physical therapist assistant, you are treating a 3-year-old child who is afflicted with cystic fibrosis. You should know that the primary area affected by this disease is the:
A. liver
B. kidneys
C. heart
D. pancreas

28. As a physical therapist assistant, you are testing the hip lateral rotation muscle strength of a 45-year-old patient who was involved in an automobile accident. The origin of the quadratus femoris is the external border of the ischial tuberosity. The insertion of this muscle is:
A. posterior surface of neck of femur
B. proximal part of linea quadrata of femur
C. superior border of greater trochanter of femur
D. medial surface of greater trochanter

29. You are treating a patient with a lesion of the inferior gluteal nerve. Which of the following motions would be the most affected?
A. hip extension
B. hip adduction
C. hip abduction
D. hip flexion

30. All of the following complications are results of a fracture except:
A. crush syndrome
B. contracture
C. loss of muscle strength
D. fat embolism

31. The spinal cord root values for the nerve that supplies the tesor fascia lata muscle is:
A. L2, L3, S5
B. L4, L5, S1
C. L1, L2, L3
D. S1, S3, S4

32. A 25-year-old woman involved in a car accident has been diagnosed with a fracture of the right clavicle. The patient complains of pain, swelling, numbness, and weakness in the right upper extremity. As a physical therapist assistant, you should suspect that one of the possible causes for these symptoms could be:
A. Von Recklinghausen's Syndrome
B. thoracic outlet syndrome
C. carpal tunnel syndrome
D. Volkmann's Syndrome

33. You are treating a patient with a strained deltoid ligament. The patient is complaining of pain, numbness, and a tingling sensation. Which of the following ligaments is most likely involved in causing these symptoms?
A. medial collateral ligament of the ankle
B. lateral collateral ligament of the knee
C. medial collateral ligament of the knee
D. lateral collateral ligament of the ankle

34. All of the following are symptoms of AIDS except:
A. general weakness
B. skin irritation
C. pulmonary complications
D. all of the above are symtoms of AIDS

35. As a physical therapist assistant working in an outpatient clinic, you are treating a patient who has sustained a sciatic nerve injury. After conducting several tests, you find that the patient has motor loss:
A. in the foot and entire leg
B. in the pelvis and hip
C. in the pelvis and lumbar spine
D. in the posterior thigh, leg, and foot

36. While working in an acute care unit as a physical therapist assistant, you receive an order to treat a 25-year-old male who has been involved in an automobile accident. He has been diagnosed with a closed head injury. On the referral, it is listed that the patient has been diagnosed as HIV+. You do not wish to treat this patient because of the possibility of contracting AIDS. You tell your supervisor how you feel, but the supervisor tells you that you should continue treatment. What would be an appropriate response?
A. treat the patient
B. treat the patient, but report the incident to the physical therapy director
C. ask one of your co-workers to treat the patient
D. refuse to treat the patient, but report the incident to the physical therapy director

37. You are treating a 20-year-old man who sustained a shoulder injury while playing baseball. On his physical therapy referral you see that the patient has a tear in the supraspinatus muscle. What is the most appropriate test to use on this patient?
A. drop-arm test
B. Yergason Test
C. Tinel Sign
D. Phalen's Test

38. You are treating a 45-year-old male who has sustained a cerebral vascular accident. You want to improve trunk control, as the patient shows poor control of the trunk. Which of the following PNF techniques would you use?
A. hold-relax
B. rhythmic initiation
C. tonic holding
D. cocontraction

39. Spina bifida is one of the more common congential disorders. Clinical findings of this birth defect might include all of the following except:
A. normal lamina and spinous processes of one or more vertebrae
B. incomplete closure of the neural plate
C. severe paralysis
D. excretory dysfunctions

40. You are treating a 32-year-old male with a left above knee amputation who is full weight bearing, and you are giving instructions on the proper stair climbing method for ascending while using axillary crutches. Which of the following climbing sequences is correct for this patient?
A. right lower extremity up, left lower extremity up, right crutch up, left crutch up
B. left lower extremity up, right lower extremity up, left crutch up, right crutch up
C. right lower extremity up, left lower extremity up, left crutch up, right crutch up
D. left lower extremity up, right lower extremity up, right crutch up, left crutch up

41. You are treating a patient who has suffered a second degree burn of the shoulder axilla. As a physical therapist assistant, you should know that the proper position for this to prevent contraction or deformity is:
A. shoulder extension and adduction
B. shoulder extension and abduction
C. shoulder flexion and abduction
D. shoulder flexion and external rotation

42. A 55-year-old male with diabetes is referred to you for therapy following an above knee left lower extremity amputation as a result of poor circulation. As the patient's physical therapist assistant, you are observing the patient and reviewing the long term goals. Which of the following are valid long term goals for this patient?
A. independent in all ambulation and self-care activities
B. independent in bed mobility and transfer
C. prevent the development of joint contractures
D. maintain or regain strength in the affected lower extremity

43. You are treating a 45-year-old patient with a chronic heart disease. Before doing exercises, it is important to do warm-up activities. These activities promote the adjustments that the body must make before doing strenuous activity. Specifically, the warm-up period:
A. decreases venous return
B. decreases need for oxygen
C. increases muscle temperature
D. increases heart rate to within 40 beats per minute of target heart rate

44. What is the average resting heart rate for infants?
A. 126 for girls, 135 for boys
B. 220 minus infants age
C. 180 for girls, 190 for boys
D. the average resting heart rate for infants is the same as for adults

45. A 25-year-old female suffered a subluxation of the radial head as a result of a fall taken while walking her dog. Given what you know about this condition, commonly known as "pushed elbow", what clinical findings would you expect to see in this patient?
A. the radial head is pushed distally in the annular ligament
B. occurs as a result of a fall on the shoulder
C. occurs as a result of a fall on the outstretched hand
D. all of the above are common clinical findings

46. During isometric exercises, you can expect to find all of the following occurrences except:
A. muscle contracts without a change in the length
B. no visible joint motion
C. strength developing at position exercise is performed
D. muscle contracts with change in the length

47. All of the following are typical soft-tissue lesions except:
A. sprain
B. fracture
C. strain
D. subluxation

48. When treating a patient who has recently undergone an amputation, what things must you be sure to check for to be certain that the prosthesis has been properly fitted?
A. discoloration
B. proper weight bearing
C. height of the posterior wall of the socket
D. all of the above

49. As a physical therapist assistant, you are treating a patient with an acute tendon rupture of the shoulder. During the acute stage, it is normal to observe pain and limited movement in the affected area. Which of the following are possible causes of this problem?
A. edema
B. muscle spasm
C. irritating chemicals
D. all of the above

50. A 72-year-old male patient is referred to you for physical therapy treatment after having a fall and fracturing his hip. The patient had an open reduction and internal fixation of the hip. In order to achieve normal hip functioning, all of the following goals must be accomplished except:
A. no pain in the hip
B. stable extremity for weight bearing
C. full range of motion and strength
D. use of an assistive device

51. What are typical treatment goals for the acute stage of bursitis?
A. control the amount of pain
B. control edema
C. maintain soft-tissue and joint mobility
D. all of the above

52. A 16-year-old patient sustained an acute sprain and partial tear of the ligaments in his knee while playing volleyball. Which of the following methods of treatment would be most appropriate for this patient?
A. rest
B. joint protection
C. gentle exercises
D. all of the above are appropriate

53. All of the following are typical causes of chondromalacia patellae except:
A. virus
B. prolonged or repeated stress
C. surgery
D. trauma

54. You are treating a 65-year-old male patient who is suffering from rheumatoid arthritis. As a physical therapist assistant, you know that rheumatoid arthritis is:
A. a connective tissue disease
B. degenerative disorder of the muscles
C. degenerative disorder of the articular cartilage
D. none of the above

55. While you are treating a patient who has sustained a fracture of the tibia, during the immobilization period you should expect to find all of the following except:
A. muscle atrophy
B. increased circulation
C. contracture formation
D. decreased circulation

56. You are treating a 38-year-old woman suffering from multiple sclerosis. According to the initial evaluation, the patient shows many abnormalities. Which of the following symptoms should you expect to find in a person diagnosed with multiple sclerosis?
A. motor weakness
B. diplopia
C. ataxic gait
D. all of the above

57. While treating a patient with a denervated muscle, it is important to consider all of the following factors except:
A. frequency
B. patient's age
C. duration
D. intensity

58. Which of the following muscles causes compression and downward translation of the humerus?
A. infraspinatus
B. teres minor
C. subscapularis
D. all of the above

59. A 25-year-old female patient has suffered a severe head injury during a car accident. During the therapist's initial evaluation, the family begins to question you on the rate and amount of recovery they can expect from the patient. You should tell the family that the majority of recovery will take place:
A. within the first month
B. within the first 3 months
C. within the first 6 months
D. within the first year

60. A patient who has sustained an anterior shoulder dislocation as a result of a fall has been referred to you for physical therapy. You have read the diagnosis but have not yet spoken to the patient regarding the injury. You should know from the diagnosis that this type of dislocation is caused by:
A. excessive internal rotation with abduction of the shoulder
B. excessive external rotation with adduction of the shoulder
C. excessive external rotation with abduction of the shoulder
D. excessive internal rotation with adduction of the shoulder

61. Which of the following is the correct definition for a second-degree burn?
A. damage through the dermal layer
B. damage to the epidermal layer
C. damage to the epidermal and part of dermal layer
D. none of the above are correct definitions of second-degree burns

62. You are treating a 32-year-old patient who has recently sprained his ankle. You are instructed to use cryotherapy as the form of treatment. Which of the following is an effect of cryotherapy?
A. increase in local metabolism
B. increase in local perspiration
C. promotion of muscle relaxation
D. decrease in local metabolism

63. Carpal tunnel syndrome involves intrinsic muscles of the thenar eminence and lumbricals. Which of the following nerves are involved with this condition?
A. ulnar nerve
B. radial nerve
C. median nerve
D. thoracic nerve

64. You are treating a patient with a peripheral vascular disease. You are ordered by the physician to use diathermy. You should be aware that the most appropriate length of treatment using diathermy for this condition is:
A. 5 minutes
B. 5 to 10 minutes
C. 20 to 30 minutes
D. 30 to 40 minutes

65. Asthma is an obstructive lung disease most often seen in a young patient. All of the following are accurate clinical pictures of this affliction except:
A. rounded shoulders
B. exocrine gland dysfunction
C. abnormal breathing pattern
D. chronic fatigue

66. Which of the following joints can you classify as hinge joints?
A. knee
B. hip
C. shoulder
D. wrist

67. A patient who has sustained a right knee sprain is referred to you for physical therapy. After several weeks of treatment, the patient still complains of pain. You decide to use ultrasound to treat this patient. What wattage would you use to increase the nerve conduction velocity?
A. 1 Watt/ cm2
B. 1.5 Watt/ cm2
C. 3 Watt/ cm2
D. both A and B are acceptable wattages

68. A 10-year-old child is being treated for lumbar lordosis. Which of the following spinal orthoses would you use to treat this problem?
A. Tyler's brace
B. Oswald's brace
C. Milwaukee brace
D. William's brace

69. A 13-year-old boy injured his knee playing soccer and requires physical therapy. During the treatment, you find instability of the knee. Which of the following ligaments provides anterior-posterior stability?
A. posterior cruciate ligament
B. anterior cruciate ligament
C. medial collateral ligament
D. both A and B

70. You are doing the daily documentation for your home health care patient who is recovering from stroke. You observe that the patient is having a good day and seems happy. In which section of the "SOAP" note would you place this entry?
A. objective
B. subjective
C. assessment
D. plan

71. Scoliosis is a spinal defect which causes postural deformity. In order to measure the amount of spinal curvature, there are many types of tests available. Which of the following is a type of measurement test of spinal curvature?
A. Master's test
B. Kerring test
C. Cobb method
D. Hoover method

72. While teaching a patient breathing excercises for her home program, what should you tell the patient to avoid doing?
A. do not force expiration
B. do not take a prolonged expiration
C. do not initiate inspiration with the upper chest
D. all of the above

73. After an amputation, there are many complications and problems that a patient must overcome. One of the most common psychological problems is that the patient continues to feel the removed extremity even though it is no longer there. This condition is known as:
A. myodesis
B. phantom limb
C. stubbies
D. none of the above

74. You are treating a 75-year-old female who sustained a right hip fracture. She is currently full weight bearing and her upper extremity strength is grossly fair plus. Which assistive device would be most appropriate for this patient?
A. wheeled walker
B. large base support quad cane
C. small base support quad cane
D. crutches

75. Multiple sclerosis is a demyelinating disease of the central nervous system that is not yet curable. This disease is most often seen in:
A. young adult females
B. young adult males
C. children
D. none of the above

76. You are treating a 30-year-old female patient who has chronic lower back pain. The attending physician has ordered ultrasound treatment; however, because the patient is 4 months pregnant, you know that ultrasound should not be used. The appropriate response in this situation is to:
A. continue treatment as ordered
B. use hot packs instead of ultrasound
C. call the doctor and discuss the situation
D. tell the patient that the doctor made a mistake and you cannot use ultrasound

77. When you are working with geriatric patients, it is important to keep in mind that certain exercises don't need to be focused on. All of the following exercises should *not* be focused on with geriatric patients except:
A. hip flexion
B. hip extension
C. knee extension
D. knee flexion

78. The foot is a part of the body that provides stability as well as mobility of the lower extremity. There are three parts of the foot: the hindfoot, the midfoot, and the forefoot. Which of the following bones belong to the midfoot?
A. talus, cuboid, and navicular
B. three cuneiforms, talus, and cuboid
C. navicular, cuboid, and three cuneiforms
D. five metatarsals, navicular, and cuboid

79. A patient who is 3 days status post total knee replacement is receiving treatment from you. The physician has ordered the use of continuous passive motion as a treatment method. One of the advantages of this type of treatment is:
A. decrease contracture formation
B. decrease postoperative pain
C. decrease joint effusion
D. all of the above

80. All of the following are characteristics of agnosia except:
A. simultagnosia
B. prosopagnosia
C. ideognosia
D. color agnosia

81. There are many deformities related to rheumatoid arthritis. One of these deformities is known as a boutonniere deformity. The characteristics of this affliction are:
A. DIP hyperextension with PIP flexion
B. DIP flexion with PIP hyperextension
C. DIP extension with PIP flexion
D. DIP flexion with PIP extension

82. An 18-year-old patient with a fractured left femur is non-weight bearing and needs physical therapy. You decide to use axillary crutches for gait training. What is the appropriate method for measuring these crutches?
A. while standing, the crutches should be 2 inches below the axilla and the distal end of the crutch should be 2 inches lateral and 6 inches anterior to the foot
B. while standing, the crutches should be 6 inches below the axilla and the distal end of the crutch should be 4 inches lateral and 4 inches anterior to the foot
C. while standing, the crutches should be directly under the axilla and the distal end of the crutch should be 3 inches lateral and 2 inches anterior to the foot
D. while standing, the crutches should be 4 inches below the axilla and the distal end of the crutch should be 4 inches lateral and 4 inches anterior to the foot.

83. You are a home health care therapist assistant visiting your patient at the scheduled time and date. When you arrive at the patient's home, you find that a nurse's aide has just begun to prepare the patient for a bath. What is the most appropriate response?
A. tell the nurse's aide to stop her activities and wait until you have finished your treatment
B. tell the patient that you can't wait for him and you will reschedule for another day
C. call your supervisor and explain the problem
D. tell the patient that they will have to miss this visit and you will be back for the next regularly scheduled visit

84. A 65-year-old male has suffered a stroke and needs physical therapy. During gait training, the patient has difficulty raising his heel during toe off. Which of the following muscles need to be strengthened to correct this gait deviation?
A. anterior tibialis
B. quadriceps
C. gastroc-soleus
D. rectus femoris

85. A 55-year-old female has been referred for physical therapy. She shows the following symptoms: mutilans type deformity, hammer toes, exostoses, and pannus. Based on this information, this patient is probably suffering from:
A. Parkinson's disease
B. rheumatoid arthritis
C. multiple sclerosis
D. arthritis

86. Which of the following conditions are not important when observing gait?
A. area in which the patient will walk
B. previous selection of joint or segment to be observed
C. select a plane observation
D. patient's weight

87. Parkinson's disease is a progressive disease which affects males more often than females. What are the major central nervous system structures involved in this disease?
A. spinal cord
B. pons
C. thalamus
D. none of the above

88. While treating patients with total hip replacements, during the first few weeks following the operation it is important to avoid all of the following actions except:
A. isometric exercises
B. hip flexion beyond 45 degrees
C. hip adduction across the midline
D. avoid excessive bending of the trunk over the hip

89. While you are treating a patient who has sustained a head injury while playing football, you observe that the patient has a tendency to cross the midline during his gait. As a physical therapist assistant, you can classify this gait pattern as:
A. spastic
B. scissor
C. gluteal
D. tabetic

90. You want to check if there is a tear in the supraspinatus muscles. Which of the following would be the most appropriate test to determine this?
A. apprehension test
B. Adson test
C. drop arm test
D. Phalen's test

91. Which of the following definitions best describe a complete lesion in a spinal cord injury?
A. some sensory or motor function below the level of the lesion
B. no motor function below the level of the lesion
C. no sensory or motor function below the level of the lesion
D. none of the above

92. Physical therapist assistants can do all of the following except:
A. administer therapeutic modalities
B. measure muscle strength
C. modify treatment plan
D. measure range of motion

93. When beginning home health care for a patient, what is the most important factor to consider?
A. diagnosis
B. home-bound status
C. patient's motivation
D. patient's age

94. All of the following are valid uses of a SOAP note except:
A. research
B. quality assurance
C. scheduling
D. communication

95. You are a physical therapist assistant checking the range of motion of the right knee of a patient who underwent total knee replacement surgery. In what portion of the SOAP note would you enter the results of this test?
A. objective
B. subjective
C. assessment
D. plan

96. While writing the objective section of a SOAP note regarding a patient's gait, all of the following are necessary components of the entry except:
A. weight bearing status
B. equipment needed
C. patient's motivation
D. type of assistance

97. Which of the following entries belongs in the assessment section of a SOAP note?
A. independent transfers on/off toilet, supine to sit, sit to stand, chair to bed. Patient is safe for activity of daily living at home within 3 weeks
B. transfers: sit to stand, wheelchair to mat with moderate assist of 1. Supine to sit with minimal assist of 1 to move patient's right lower extremity
C. patient complaining of severe pain with active range of motion exercises
D. active range of motion of right knee 30 to 45 degrees. All other joints within normal limits

98. All of the following are typical symptoms for myasthenia gravis except:
A. limb weakness
B. dysarthria
C. dysphasia
D. hemiplegia

99. You are treating a patient 3 days status post stroke with left side flaccid. You are instructed by the attending physical therapist to use a sling in order to:
A. correct the cause of the subluxation
B. prevent additional subluxation
C. improve muscle strength
D. facilitate movement patterns

100. In research, which term describes a test that gives the same results every time?
A. validity
B. reliability
C. significance
D. none of the above

Chapter 14
Helpful Hints

1. Plan a schedule for studying each section.

2. Don't study hard the night before the test. Get a good night's sleep.

3. Look on a map to determine exactly how to get to the test site.

4. Know the room number and how to get to it.

5. Make sure you are at the test site at least 45 minutes before it starts.

6. Bring a watch to the exam.

7. Have 2 or 3 extra pencils with an eraser.

8. Try to give yourself space when choosing a seat.

9. Relax! Be confident that you have done the best you could to prepare for the test.

Answer Keys

Chapter 8
Multiple Choice Phrases

1. A
2. C
3. C
4. C
5. B
6. D
7. A
8. D
9. D
10. D
11. B
12. A
13. C
14. A
15. D
16. D
17. D
18. C
19. B
20. A
21. B
22. D
23. B
24. D
25. B
26. D
27. C
28. D
29. A
30. D

Chapter 9
Prefixes and Suffixes

1. motion, not moving
2. appear, to be seen again
3. practice, improper or negligent treatment of a patient by a physician
4. restrict, tending to confine or restrain
5. accurate, not accurately; incorrectly
6. pressure, to provide resistance against a patient's movement
7. initial, to cause to begin
8. relevant, not relevant; not important
9. immerse, capable of being put completely in water without suffering damage
10. instruct, teaching; giving knowledge
11. reduce, the act of process of lessening something
12. judge, making decisions
13. adolescent, a child between the ages of 10 and 12; before adolescence
14. support, without support
15. minimum, reduce to the smallest possible amount
16. trust, feeling or showing doubt
17. objective, making decisions without any emotions
18. inflammatory, pertaining to a substance or procedure that counteracts or reduces inflammation
19. proper, not properly; incorrectly
20. weak, the state of being weak; not strong
21. typical, not typical; unusual
22. pressure, to release from pressure
23. normal, less than or below normal
24. tester, inter: same test done by two or more therapists
25. tester, intra: same test done by one therapist
26. legible, not legible; not able to read
27. operate, occurring after surgery
28. diagnose, diagnosed incorrectly
29. essential, not essential; not necessary
30. therapy, having healing or curative powers

Chapter 10
English Words

(p. 52)
1. unconscious 2. complications 3. impairment 4. shortness of breath 5. harmful 6. sustained injury 7. tenderness 8. tight 9. deviation 10. obese

(p. 55)
1. allow for 2. in and above 3. course of action 4. associated with 5. out of proportion 6. results in 7. in order to

(p. 47)
1. severe 2. mild 3. moderate; mild; severe 4. chronic 5. acute

(p. 46)
1. duration 2. immediate 3. prolong 4. short-term 5. long-term 6. consistently 7. frequency 8. occasionally

(p. 64)
1. supine 2. absent 3. proper 4. willingness 5. strength 6. affect 7. maintaining 8. evident 9. achieve 10. regarding 11. potential

(p. 53)
1. HMOs 2. discharged 3. litigation 4. in-patient 5. entries 6. recording 7. out-patient 8. document

(p. 56)
1. statistical significance 2. significant 3. reliable 4. valid 5. clinical

(p. 45)
1. entire 2. majority 3. more 4. maximal 5. increased 6. sufficient 7. partially 8. fully 9. amount 10. decrease 11. excessive 12. minimum 13. additional 14. most 15. certain 16. normal 17. total

(p. 59)
1. conducting 2. emphasis 3. delay 4. elect 5. compensate for 6. integrate 7. provide 8. apply 9. utilize

(p. 50)
1. techniques 2. implement 3. touch 4. place 5. resistance 6. treatment 7. task 8. stabilize 9. stationary 10. methods 11. training 12. pressure 13. apply 14. stretching 15. tension

(p. 57)
1. vary 2. improve 3. variety 4. review 5. modified

(p. 62)
1. benefits 2. facilitate 3. support 4. progress

(p. 43)
1. determine 2. measure 3. diagnosis 4. objectivity 5. evaluates 6. criteria
7. screening 8. identify 9. goals 10. note 11. findings 12. results

(p. 61)
1. inhibited 2. disregard 3. disrupted 4. failure to 5. restrict 6. diminish 7. eliminating

(p. 63)
1. 3 weeks status post 2. secreting 3. precautions 4. vital signs 5. intervention 6. drain
7. digits 8. ipsilateral 9. internal 10. post-operative 11. contraindicated
12. extremities; extremities 13. modalities 14. external

(p. 48)
1. ascending 2. descending 3. rhythm 4. kneel 5. reflex 6. immersing 7. ROM
8. elevated 9. movable; immovable 10. repetitions 11. lower 12. motion 13. raise

(p. 60)
1. considered 2. detect 3. expect 4. unknown 5. comprehends 6. sense 7. assume

(p. 44)
1. symptoms 2. exhibit 3. background 4. condition 5. history of 6. behavior 7. signs
8. appears 9. characteristic 10. demonstrate 11. denotes

(p. 49)
1. after 2. initial 3. before 4. between 5. during 6. further 7. behind 8. prior to
9. position

(p. 51)
1. fracture 2. strain 3. cough 4. burns 5. pain 6. sprained 7. swelling 8. accidents
9. rupture 10. deep laceration 11. weakness

(p. 58)
1. prevent 2. assist 3. elicit 4. discuss 5. dismiss 6. performing 7. instruct
8. continued 9. attempt 10. obtain

(p. 54)
1. acceptable 2. appropriate 3. accurate 4. necessary 5. viable 6. able 7. practical
8. essential 9. effective

Chapter 12
PT Practice Exam

1. B
2. B
3. D
4. A
5. D
6. A
7. A
8. B
9. C
10. A
11. B
12. C
13. A
14. C
15. A
16. D
17. C
18. D
19. C
20. A
21. D
22. C
23. A
24. B
25. D
26. A
27. A
28. B
29. A
30. A
31. A
32. D
33. C
34. C
35. B
36. C
37. D
38. A
39. C
40. C
41. D
42. D
43. D
44. D
45. D
46. D
47. B
48. A
49. B
50. C
51. C
52. D
53. C
54. D
55. B
56. D
57. C
58. C
59. D
60. A
61. A
62. B
63. D
64. A
65. C
66. B
67. A
68. C
69. C
70. D
71. D
72. D
73. C
74. A
75. D
76. C
77. B
78. D
79. C
80. A
81. D
82. D
83. C
84. A
85. A
86. A
87. A
88. B
89. A
90. C
91. B
92. B
93. C
94. A
95. D
96. C
97. B
98. B
99. A
100. B

Chapter 13
PTA Practice Exam

1. C
2. B
3. D
4. A
5. D
6. C
7. D
8. A
9. B
10. B
11. A
12. C
13. D
14. B
15. A
16. A
17. A
18. B
19. A
20. C
21. D
22. D
23. B
24. C
25. C
26. C
27. D
28. B
29. A
30. A
31. B
32. B
33. A
34. D
35. D
36. D
37. A
38. B
39. A
40. A
41. C
42. A
43. C
44. A
45. C
46. D
47. B
48. D
49. D
50. D
51. D
52. D
53. A
54. A
55. B
56. D
57. B
58. D
59. C
60. C
61. C
62. D
63. C
64. C
65. B
66. A
67. C
68. D
69. D
70. B
71. C
72. D
73. B
74. A
75. A
76. C
77. A
78. C
79. D
80. C
81. C
82. A
83. B
84. C
85. B
86. D
87. D
88. A
89. B
90. C
91. C
92. C
93. B
94. C
95. A
96. C
97. A
98. D
99. B
100. B

Answer Sheet

	A	B	C	D
1.	O	O	O	O
2.	O	O	O	O
3.	O	O	O	O
4.	O	O	O	O
5.	O	O	O	O
6.	O	O	O	O
7.	O	O	O	O
8.	O	O	O	O
9.	O	O	O	O
10.	O	O	O	O
11.	O	O	O	O
12.	O	O	O	O
13.	O	O	O	O
14.	O	O	O	O
15.	O	O	O	O
16.	O	O	O	O
17.	O	O	O	O
18.	O	O	O	O
19.	O	O	O	O
20.	O	O	O	O
21.	O	O	O	O
22.	O	O	O	O
23.	O	O	O	O
24.	O	O	O	O
25.	O	O	O	O
26.	O	O	O	O
27.	O	O	O	O
28.	O	O	O	O
29.	O	O	O	O
30.	O	O	O	O
31.	O	O	O	O
32.	O	O	O	O
33.	O	O	O	O
34.	O	O	O	O
35.	O	O	O	O
36.	O	O	O	O
37.	O	O	O	O
38.	O	O	O	O
39.	O	O	O	O
40.	O	O	O	O
41.	O	O	O	O
42.	O	O	O	O
43.	O	O	O	O
44.	O	O	O	O
45.	O	O	O	O
46.	O	O	O	O
47.	O	O	O	O
48.	O	O	O	O
49.	O	O	O	O
50.	O	O	O	O
51.	O	O	O	O
52.	O	O	O	O
53.	O	O	O	O
54.	O	O	O	O
55.	O	O	O	O
56.	O	O	O	O
57.	O	O	O	O
58.	O	O	O	O
59.	O	O	O	O
60.	O	O	O	O
61.	O	O	O	O
62.	O	O	O	O
63.	O	O	O	O
64.	O	O	O	O
65.	O	O	O	O
66.	O	O	O	O
67.	O	O	O	O
68.	O	O	O	O
69.	O	O	O	O
70.	O	O	O	O
71.	O	O	O	O
72.	O	O	O	O
73.	O	O	O	O
74.	O	O	O	O
75.	O	O	O	O
76.	O	O	O	O
77.	O	O	O	O
78.	O	O	O	O
79.	O	O	O	O
80.	O	O	O	O
81.	O	O	O	O
82.	O	O	O	O
83.	O	O	O	O
84.	O	O	O	O
85.	O	O	O	O
86.	O	O	O	O
87.	O	O	O	O
88.	O	O	O	O
89.	O	O	O	O
90.	O	O	O	O
91.	O	O	O	O
92.	O	O	O	O
93.	O	O	O	O
94.	O	O	O	O
95.	O	O	O	O
96.	O	O	O	O
97.	O	O	O	O
98.	O	O	O	O
99.	O	O	O	O
100.	O	O	O	O

ERRATA

Korzeniowska, I., Schnoll, R., & Tomaszkiewicz, A. (1995). ***PT exam review: The essential guide for the foreign-trained physical therapist.*** **Thorofare, NJ: SLACK Incorporated.**

The following is a list of corrections to text and answers that were incorrectly printed.

Page 94, question 9
Answer B should read:
passive patient participation

Page 99, question 38
Answer B should read:
rhythmic stabilization

Page 105, question 77
The second sentence of the question should read:
All of the following exercises should be focused on with geriatric patients except:

Page 119, PTA Practice Exam Answer Key

9.	A
36.	A
67.	D
81.	A

SLACK Incorporated, 6900 Grove Road, Thorofare, NJ 08086-9447
Phone: 609-848-1000; Fax: 609-853-5991